OCR →

Healing the Dying

Healing
the Dying

MELODIE OLSON, PhD, RN
College of Nursing
Medical University of South Carolina
Charleston, South Carolina

Delmar Publishers

 I(T)P™

An International Thomson Publishing Company

Albany • Bonn • Boston • Cincinnati • Detroit • London
Madrid • Melbourne • Mexico City • New York • Pacific Grove
Paris • San Francisco • Singapore • Tokyo • Toronto • Washington

NOTICE TO THE READER

Cover Design: Spiral Design
Cover Illustration: Kirsten Soderlind

Delmar Staff
Senior Acquisitions Editor: Bill Burgower
Assistant Editor: Hilary Schrauf
Senior Project Editor: Judith Boyd Nelson
Production Coordinator: Barbara A. Bullock
Art and Design Coordinator: Timothy J. Conners

COPYRIGHT © 1997
By Delmar Publishers
a division of International Thomson Publishing Inc.

The ITP logo is a trademark under license.

Printed in the United States of America

For more information, contact:

Delmar Publishers
3 Columbia Circle, Box 15015
Albany, New York 12212-5015

International Thomson Publishing Europe
Berkshire House 168-173
High Holborn
London, WC1V 7AA
England

Thomas Nelson Australia
102 Dodds Street
South Melbourne, 3205
Victoria, Australia

Nelson Canada
1120 Birchmount Road
Scarborough, Ontario
Canada, M1K 5G4

International Thomson Editores
Campos Eliseos 385, Piso 7
Col Polanco
11560 Mexico D F Mexico

International Thomson Publishing GmbH
Konigswinterer Strasse 418
53227 Bonn
Germany

International Thomson Publishing Asia
221 Henderson Road
#05-10 Henderson Building
Singapore 0315

International Thomson Publishing—Japan
Hirakawacho Kyowa Building, 3F
2-2-1 Hirakawacho
Chiyoda-ku, Tokyo 102
Japan

1 2 3 4 5 6 7 8 9 10 XXX 02 01 00 99 98 97 96

Library of Congress Cataloging-in-Publication Data

Olson, Melodie
   Healing the dying / Melodie Olson.
      p.   cm. — (Nurse as healer series)
   Includes bibliographical references and index.
   ISBN 0-8273-6603-5
   1. Terminal care.   2. Death.   I. Title.   II. Series.
   [DNLM: 1. Terminal Care — methods — nurses' instruction.
   2. Palliative Treatment — nursing.   3. Attitude to Death.   4. Social
   Support.   WY 152 052h 1996]
   RT87.T45047   1997
   362.1'75 — dc20
   DNLM/DLC
   for Library of Congress   95-45489
                                                                                    CIP

INTRODUCTION
TO NURSE AS
HEALER SERIES

LYNN KEEGAN, PhD, RN, Series Editor

Associate Professor, School of Nursing,
University of Texas Health Science Center at San Antonio
San Antonio, Texas
and Director of BodyMind Systems, Temple, Texas

To nurse means to care for or to nurture with compassion. Most nurses begin their formal education with this ideal. Many nurses retain this orientation after graduation, and some manage their entire careers under this guiding principle of caring. Many of us, however, tend to forget this ideal in the hectic pace of our professional and personal lives. We may become discouraged and feel a sense of burnout.

Throughout the past decade I have spoken at many conferences with thousands of nurses. Their experience of frustration and failure is quite common. These nurses feel themselves spread as pawns across a health care system too large to control or understand. In part, this may be because they have forgotten their true roles as nurse-healers.

When individuals redirect their personal vision and empower themselves, an entire pattern may begin to change. And so it is now with the nursing profession. Most of us conceptualize nursing as much more than a vocation. We are greater than our individual roles as scientists, specialists, or care deliverers. We currently search for a name to put on our new conception of the empowered nurse. The recently introduced term *nurse-healer* aptly describes the qualities of an increasing number of clinicians, educators, administrators, and nurse practitioners. Today all nurses are awakening to the realization that they have the potential for healing.

It is my feeling that most nurses, when awakened and guided to develop their own healing potential, will function both as nurses and healers. Thus, the concept of nurse as healer is born. When nurses realize they have the ability to evoke others' healing, as well as care for them, a shift of consciousness begins to occur. As individual awareness and changes in skill building occur, a collective understanding of this new concept emerges. This knowledge, along with a shift in attitudes and new kinds of behavior, allows empowered nurses to renew themselves in an expanded role. The Nurse As Healer Series is born out of the belief that nurses are ready to embrace guidance that inspires them in their journeys of empowerment. Each book in the series may stand alone or be used in complementary fashion with other books. I hope and believe that information herein will strengthen you both personally and professionally, and provide you with the help and confidence to embark upon the path of nurse-healer.

Titles in the Nurse As Healer Series:

Healing Touch: A Resource for Health Care Professionals

Healing Life's Crises: A Guide for Nurses

The Nurse's Meditative Journal

Healing Nutrition

Healing the Dying

Awareness in Healing

Creative Imagery in Nursing

DEDICATION

For Dad, Evelyn, and Charles, who live well.

C O N T E N T S

Preface, *xv*
Acknowledgments, *xvii*

Part 1 **THE SOCIOLOGY OF DEATH, 1**

    Chapter 1 **What Does It Mean to Heal the Dying?,**
                 3
                 Dying Healed, 3
                 Healing as Relationship, 4
                 Palliative Care and Healing, 7
                 Summary, 8
                 References, 8

    Chapter 2 **The Sociology of Death: Patterns and**
                 Values, 9
                 The Relationship of Death and Society, 9
                   Language and Symbols, 9
                   Art, 11
                   Ritual, 12
                 Mortality Through the Ages, 14
                   Mortality Before the Industrial
                   Revolution, 15
                   From the Industrial Revolution to World
                   War II, 16
                   Post World War II, 16
                   Death at Present, 19
                 Peaceful Death: Letting Go, 20
                 Summary, 22
                 References, 22

Chapter 3   ***Theories Related to Dying, Healing, 25***

The Usefulness of Theory, 25

Grief Theory, 26
Definitions, 26
Developmental Theory, 27
Characteristics of Grief, 28
Consequences of Grief, 29

Family Theory, 31
Types of Families, 32
Family Theories, 32
Developmental Family Theory, 33
Structural/Functional Family Theory, 34
Family Systems Theory, 35
Grief and Family, 36

Self-Transcendence, 39
Summary, 41

References, 42

Part 2   **COMFORT OF THE DYING INDIVIDUAL, 45**

Chapter 4   ***Goals for Comfort in Dying, 47***

Comfort Defined, 47

Quality of Life, 48

Assessment, 50

Comfort for the Whole Person, 53
Presence, 53
Surveillance and Safety, 54
Choice, 54
Environment, 55

Specific Areas of Comfort Needs, 56
Sleep, 56
Movement, 60
Touch, 64
Summary, 66

References, 66

Chapter 5   ***Pain Management, 69***

The Problem, 69

Pain Defined, 70

Assessment, 72
Interview, 72

Rating Scales, 73
A Child's Pain, 76

Theories of Pain, 77
Transmission of Pain, 77
Perception of Pain, 79

Pharmacologic Treatment of Pain, 79
Additives and Adjuvants, 80
Complications, 80
Timing of Administration, 82
Methods of Administration, 82

Nonpharmacologic Treatment of Pain, 85
Surgical Intervention, 86
Acupuncture, 86
Noninvasive Pain Control, 86
Electrical Stimulation, 87
Physical Stimulation, 88
Therapeutic Touch (TT), 89
Behavioral/Cognitive Interventions, 90

Creative Arts, 92

Summary, 93

References, 93

**Chapter 6   Care of the Person Who Is Frightened,
95**

The Problem, 95

Fear, 96

Anxiety, 98

Coping, 98

Assessment, 101

Communication, 102
Taking In Information, 105
Responding, 106

Support Groups, 108

Other Techniques for Reduction of Fear and
Anxiety, 110
Visualization, 111
Humor, 113
Life Review, 115

Psychiatric Illness in Dying, 116

Summary, 117

References, 118

Chapter 7 **Spirituality, 119**

The Nature of Spirituality, 119

Spiritual Development, 120

Spiritual Health, 121

Spirit and Mind, 122

Religion and Spirituality, 123

Spiritual Need and Spiritual Distress, 125
  Forgiveness, 126
  Hope, 127
  Trust, 128
  Meaning, 129

Spiritual Assessment, 130

Nursing Interventions, 131
  The Nurse, 132
  Spiritual Help for the Dying, 133

Summary, 135

References, 136

Part 3 **HELP FOR FAMILIES, 137**

Chapter 8 **Families, 139**

Goals, 139

Connecting, 141
  Truth Telling, 142
  Advocacy, 147

Legal Aspects, 149
  Advanced Directives, 151

Summary, 155

References, 155

Chapter 9 **Resources for the Dying and Their Families, 157**

The Need, 157

Finding Resources, 158

Making Referrals, 160

Government, 161
  Veteran's Administration, 162
  Research Information from the Federal Government, 163
  Local Government, 165

Nongovernmental Organizations, 165
  Hospice, 166
  Other Organizations, 171
Summary, 171
References, 172

Part 4   SPECIAL CASES, 173

Chapter 10   When Special People Die, 175

Family, 175
  Death of Parents of Adult Children, 175
  Death of Parents of Younger Children, 178
  Death of a Child, 179
  Sudden Infant Death Syndrome (SIDS), 181
  Siblings, 182
  Death of a Spouse, 183

Stigmatizing Illness, 184
  Acquired Immune Deficiency Syndrome (AIDS),
  185
  Natural History, 187

Violent Death, 190
  Suicide, 191
  Homicide, 193
  Societal Issues, 194

The Death of a Nurse, 195

Near-Death Experiences, 196

Summary, 198

References, 199

Chapter 11   Those Who Care for the Dying, 201

Caring for Dying People, 201
  One Model of Occupational Stress, 201
  Consequences of Stress for Providers of Care, 206

Changing the Environment, 208

Caring for Self, 212
  Motivation, 212
  Coping Techniques, 213

Developing the Spiritual Self, 218

Summary, 220

References, 220

Epilogue, 222

Appendix 1 Dosing Data for Pain Medications, 223

Appendix 2 Haight's Life Review and Experiencing Form,
               229

Appendix 3 Hot Lines and National Resources, 235

Index, 241

PREFACE

AIMS AND ORGANIZATION

Healing the Dying is intended to give the student and professional nurse practical guidance in the care of the dying patient, thus improving the quality of care given to the dying patient. It is intended to increase the range of choices for both the patient and the nurse so they can create an environment in which healing in its fullest sense can occur.

Healing the Dying is organized into four parts. Part 1 includes epidemiology and theories related to dying. Grief theory, family theory, and other theories are helpful in understanding the kinds of care needed. Part 2 includes concepts of comfort for the individual. Measures to control discomfort, including sleep disturbance and mobility, are covered. Pain control, fear, and spiritual distress are also included. Part 3 focuses on family and social supports, such as hospice and bereavement services. Part 4 is a special section that considers relationships between particularly vulnerable populations of patients and nurses. The patients may have a common illness, such as cancer or HIV disease, or they may share some unique event, such as a near-death experience. They may be patients who are part of the nurse's family. Self-care hints for nurses are included; e.g., how to know when to take additional time off.

Vignettes are illustrations of themes that make the theories come alive. They are useful in making content clear and in helping the reader see the relevance of ideas to care. These short stories are included in every chapter.

The English language does not have a nonspecific gender pronoun. Rather than using the awkward he/she construction to avoid appearing sexist, people are referred to as he or she. An attempt is made to alternate gender-identifying pronouns when it is possible without causing confusion in the writing. While nursing is still a predominantly female profession, men make substantial contributions to the nursing profession, and are recognized in this book.

In the appendices there are several very useful resources. Dosage tables for pain medications (from the Agency for Health Care Policy and Research) are reprinted for quick reference. There are lists of resources with addresses to help find agencies and organizations that will help with a variety of social and informational needs. A life review guide is included to guide the caregiver in leading a reminiscence session. Each of these resources is designed for easy use.

A C K N O W L E D G M E N T S

Several people have encouraged the writing of this book. Lynn Keegan had the vision to begin this incredibly useful series. The editors and staff of Delmar Publishers, particularly Bill Burgower and Debra Flis, guided the process of publishing this book with great skill. Elaine Staller and Ramita Bonadonna contributed their experience and knowledge to the content by reading drafts, suggesting changes, and encouraging the author. Thank you all!

1 | THE SOCIOLOGY OF DEATH

1 | WHAT DOES IT MEAN TO *HEAL THE DYING?*

DYING HEALED

Healing the dying sounds like an oxymoron, pulling together two contradictory thoughts. But to heal is not necessarily to cure, though that may happen during healing. To heal is to bring various levels of oneself—cellular, physical, intrapersonal, interpersonal, societal, spiritual, perhaps even cosmic—into new relationship with each other. Care of the person who is dying requires an assessment of the relationship of that person to self, others, and God, and appropriate intervention to assist with perceived deficits in these areas.

Dying *healed* means that a person has finished the business of life, said good-byes, and reached life's goals. An individual knows who he is, and has a sense of integration of self and life. The dying person recognizes that this life was his own, and no one else would have lived it the same way. His death matters to someone. Life's troubles have led to a kind of wisdom. Comfort and maybe even peace are achieved. The family has had sufficient time to grieve and to plan for the changes in the lives of its members. However, the time has not been excessive, leading to extreme emotional and physical fatigue and caregiver burnout. Control of the process of dying remains in the hands of the dying person for as long as he is able and willing to take it, fighting the good fight. When he is ready, decision making is passed to others, and a feeling of comfort results from their ministrations. Dying is perceived as a stage of life that fits into a broader philosophy giving both death and life meaning.

HEALING AS RELATIONSHIP

The notion of healing as relationship, different from curing, is an idea seen as early as Nightingale's work (1969). She wrote that the role of the nurse was to put the patient in the best possible condition so that healing could occur. Nightingale believed that the physician removed impediments to healing with surgical techniques, medications, and other medical interventions. The nurse created the appropriate environment, which was clean, airy, and cheerful, and met the nutritional requirements of the individual. After that, it was the patient who did the work. Healing came from within each person.

Nightingale's most publicized patients were those soldiers injured during the Crimean War. Like veterans of all times, their scars were evidence of physical healing. The wounds were cleaned, foreign objects and bacteria removed, gangrenous or badly mangled limbs removed by amputation, and the wound edges brought together. Healing occurred through the body's own processes of clot formation, tissue regrowth, and the immune response. These are all internal processes. The cells came into new relationship with each other. Diseases were avoided or overcome.

Scars that give evidence of healing may disrupt other relationships. A livid scar on the face may interfere with self-esteem. Disruption of self-esteem may end a love affair. An amputated limb may disrupt a profession or affect one's economic status in life. An organ that was removed may interfere with one's stamina and limit activity. Perception of the scar, or changed relationships in one's physical body, can result in bitterness, loss of friends, loss of faith, loss of meaning.

Conversely, one can view the scar with thankfulness for the healing, and begin to see past the scar. A person can begin to socialize with people for whom the scar is not a barrier. There is the possibility of achieving great satisfaction in life even with disability. Jim Abbott, born without a right hand, did not allow the lack of that hand to stop him from becoming a baseball pitcher for the Yankees. He pitched a no-hitter in the major leagues, a remarkable feat for anyone. In overcoming adversity, one develops abilities and a depth of meaning previously unknown. Friends are not limited by superficial artifacts. One learns new ways of interacting with family. A positive self-image strengthens.

Dying is a process that has many of the same characteristics as the process of scar formation. Both the scar and the dying processes cause physical change. The difference is that the scar is evidence of healing, while physical changes due to the disease process lead quite directly to the patient's death. For example, a cancerous growth may erode a necessary vascular route, causing bleeding. The skills needed to cope with the physical changes brought about by scarring or by dying are rooted in developing an awareness of the changes those processes require. Addressing those changes requires the willingness to establish and maintain a clear sense of self, and how the self relates to others.

Throughout the dying process, new relationships are forming. Perception of one's self as a dying individual could lead to loss of self-esteem, bitterness, loss of faith, loss of a sense of meaning in life. Perception of the dying person by others may also disrupt friendships and family relationships. But the dying process, like the scar, does not require that the changed relationships are negative, sad, or bitter. Persons who have been close to death but became well again often report that they have a new sense of living each moment more fully, of experiencing life with reverence, awe, and real joy. People who know they are dying sometimes capture that same spirit of satisfaction through integration of self. It is not that they want to die. A woman who was dying believed that several years prior to the current illness she had been given a new life. She had avoided death during a critical illness. Though now close to death with leukemia, she still hoped for another miracle—a postponement of death. During the first brush with death she feared the process of death. Would it hurt? What would physical symptoms be like? Is there anything that happens after the body stops breathing? None of these questions concerned her during the last stages of the leukemia. Instead, her reasons for wanting to stay a while longer on this earth were because her relationships with her grown children had become so precious she wanted to cherish them a while longer. This woman did not fear death, but lived in awe of each moment. She knew her children would be fine without her, but she had much joy in their presence. The first brush with death had gotten her beyond the fear, into a new sense of living each day fully. She sensed that when it was her time to die she would be willing to leave the family, and let go of this life peacefully.

Many people have ideas about what they want when they are dying. Often, people would like to be conscious very near the time of death, alert, and able to communicate. Dying in one's sleep is also acceptable, but not following a prolonged coma, or drawn out period of time. Most people do not want a period of suffering and/or pain, but if it is unavoidable, they would like to bear the burden with grace. People want to be treated with respect and dignity; they do not want to be abandoned by loved ones, professional people, or society. Most people recognize that there is no guarantee of a peaceful death, so they may need to develop courage (Callahan, 1993).

Mr. Bower

Mr. Bower was a 49-year-old veteran of the Korean War, who was hospitalized in a Veteran's Administration Hospital with cancer of the prostate. Because of his age, treatment was aggressive. Because he had very little support other than the Veteran's Administration, he was hospitalized for eight months before his death, with only a few weekend passes. During that time, he taught one young nurse about dying by sharing his experiences with her.

Ms. F. was a night nurse with two years of critical care experience. She had recently transferred to Mr. Bower's unit. About 3 A.M. of the second night she was there, Ms. F. found Mr. Bower smoking in the solarium. He wanted to talk. She sat with him for a few minutes, and began a pattern of relationship that lasted for the eight months they were both on the unit. Each night she was on duty, Mr. Bower waited up for her to talk more about dying. Some nights she was unable to find the time to talk, but on the nights that she did,

Mr. Bower taught Ms. F. what it was like to face death and the many choices one has to make to continue to deepen the meaning of one's life. Mr. Bower was a person who died having achieved peace and purpose. He continues to share some of his lessons in this book.

PALLIATIVE CARE AND HEALING

Healing the dying requires attention to relationship. In caring for the dying patient, the caregiver understands that the medical prognosis of the patient is limited, and care is termed *palliative.* Care focuses on quality of life rather than length of life. The World Health Organization defines palliative care as:

> The active total care of patients whose disease is not responsive to curative treatment. Control of pain, of other symptoms and of psychological, social, and spiritual problems, is paramount. The goal of palliative care is achievement of the best quality of life for patients and their families.

They add:

> Palliative care . . . affirms life and regards dying as a normal process . . . neither hastens nor postpones death, . . . provides relief from pain and other distressing symptoms, . . . integrates the psychological and spiritual aspects of care, . . . offers a support system to help patients live as actively as possible until death, . . . offers a support system to help family cope during the patient's illness and their own bereavement (Doyle, Hanks, & McDonald, 1993; World Health Organization, 1990).

The concept of healing the dying incorporates palliative care and goes beyond to nurture relationships of all kinds, to provide choices so that the dying patient can create an environment in which life can be lived to its fullest, and in which, at some point, the patient can make the choice to let go and slip into a peaceful death. The nurse or other health care provider is in full and healthy partnership with the patient during this time. Recognizing that the nurse will always feel some emotion when a patient dies opens the nurse to sharing the experience rather than denying it, dealing with often contradictory emotions. The nurse is in the environment of the dying patient, and contributes to that milieu. Making choices about care that allow the patient to live according to his wishes while following established standards of care, and caring for other patients at the same time, requires skill, knowledge, compassion, organization, and a willingness to confront one's own mortality. Many of the same issues the patient confronts in his dying are issues the nurse confronts in helping that person to live in the time allotted—issues of physical, spiritual, and psychological distress, and the need for support of different kinds. Caring for the dying patient requires caring for one's self.

SUMMARY

Healing includes new relationships between all levels of the person, leading to a feeling of well-being, safety, and peace. Healing leads to greater comfort. Healing the dying helps the dying person to a perception of life as having been meaningful. Healing the dying may occur in the presence of disease if the death ultimately is peaceful.

References

Callahan, D. (1993, July–August). *Pursuing a peaceful death* (pp. 33–38). Hasting's Center Report.

World Health Organization. (1990). *Cancer Pain Relief and Palliative Care* (Technical Report Series 804). Geneva: Author.

Doyle, D., Hanks, G. W. C., & MacDonald, N. (Eds.). (1993). *Oxford textbook of palliative medicine.* Oxford: Oxford University Press.

Nightingale, F. (1969). *Notes on nursing.* New York: Dover. (Original work published 1860)

THE SOCIOLOGY OF DEATH: PATTERNS AND VALUES

THE RELATIONSHIP OF DEATH AND SOCIETY

Societal values determine attitudes and behaviors related to death and healing. How an individual feels about death, and what actions are taken as a response to those feelings, are based in part on what society values as appropriate behavior. It is important to identify society's values, because contemporary American society relies on those values when addressing death-related social issues, and how people should behave. Those issues include extending life with technology past the time people would wish; euthanasia; abortion; capital punishment; the nature of a peaceful death; and other death-related social events. Knowing society's values helps people begin to create an environment in which each person can die peacefully. One way to begin to identify society's values in relation to death is to examine language, symbols, and rituals of death in any culture.

Language and Symbols

Language is the set of symbols by which people communicate, and by which they identify what is important and meaningful in life. A society that values esthetics highly will have a language rich in imagery and vivid description. A society that values scientific thought will have precise definitions of events, and be concise, almost terse, by comparison to the more descriptive speech.

Describing the passage of blood through the heart in some New Guinea languages takes a whole morning, as each part of each chamber is described in detail. In English, only a few sentences are necessary to list the structures passed and their functions as blood travels the short route. The use of a short, specific vocabulary for science illustrates the value the scientist places on efficiency and clarity of thought. The simpler the sentence, the more useful the concept.

The number of words a culture has for a subject, reflecting its many meanings, may be a clue to the importance of that subject for the people, and how they deal with it. In many languages, there are several words for the concept of love. Those words reflect a love of parents for children, a physical relationship with another adult, a love for God. The willingness of people to use those words and discuss the subject reflects in part how comfortable they are with the topic. Lack of words for a concept may mean that the people do not think in terms of that concept. Few words for a subject or the use of euphemism in place of those words may indicate a denial of the reality of the concept.

For some people in the United States, death is a difficult word to use. The difficulty in telling someone that he or she is dying, to discuss the impending death with family and others, or to say someone is dead at the time of the funeral reflects attitudes of the group toward death. Death becomes more tolerable if the dying one is lost, or goes to her eternal rest. Such language suggests a societal denial of death, a collusion to avoid the pain that death brings. Even death by violence may sound almost acceptable if, instead of killing someone, you waste or terminate the enemy, or put someone to sleep. It is also possible to sensitize the population to death by linking the word with other words, thus softening its meaning, as in death by chocolate, dead ahead, or you're dead right.

The language used by people not only reflects values, but changes their values in relation to the topic. Euphemisms people use are the first experiences the next generation have with the idea. Children learn that the player with the football is dead meat before they learn how it feels to miss Grandma when she dies. Society as a whole may sanction or withhold sanction for actions involving death depending on how the topic is addressed. For example, a physician may talk of *euthanasia*, a technical term, while a writer of novels terms the act a *mercy killing*. As euthanasia becomes linked with mercy, laws are more likely to change, and society seeks to find ways in which to implement the basic value of mercy.

Healing, too, reflects societal attitudes. Common usage of the term may imply religious belief to those who attend and participate in healing services at their local places of worship. The term may reflect a precise physiological pattern, as in wound healing. It is often taken to mean cure of disease, or it may mean resolution of some problem. Generally, healing is positive. Things people do to achieve healing are accepted, even when they take place outside of the common plan of action or usually approved activities, so long as they do not harm others. For example, megavitamin therapies have not been shown to be efficacious in traditional studies, but cancer patients who are dying are not prohibited from taking them if they go to herb shops or nutrition centers. Doctors generally do not prescribe the vitamins because they are not within accepted standards of medical practice.

Healing is often adopted as a positive philosophy when a society is dissatisfied with the medical care of the times. There were several periods of holistic health movements in the United States during which vitamin therapy, special baths, herbs, and other nutrients were popularized, and given status as adjuncts or aids to healing (Hamilton, 1991). Various healers such as curanderos, shamans, and religious leaders were given high status, followed or at least heard. They commonly espoused a path to a positive life—not necessarily disease free, but healthy as a whole. Almost always, interpersonal relationships were stressed by these healers.

Art

Another set of symbols that society uses to express its values and attitudes toward death and healing is art in its many forms. A life-size mural on a wall in an inner city neighborhood depicting a knife dripping blood suspended above the body of a teenager focuses attention on violence and societal tensions. The same sized mural depicting the death of Christ painted on the wall of a church focuses on religious meanings of death. A Diego Rivera larger-than-life mural on the walls of government buildings in

Mexico City makes a political statement about death. These social, religious, or political statements may contribute to an understanding of the many meanings of death.

Similarly, music that focuses on death may create a sense of sadness, as in "Ode to Billy Joe," where death occurred in youth and by choice; or as in the traditional dirge music played at the funerals of many former U.S. presidents. Music may also uplift spirits, as in traditional religious music pieces like Handel's *Messiah*. It ends with a joyous celebration of immortality— the belief that at least spiritually, there is no death.

Drama, literature, and other forms of art also reflect and change societal attitudes toward death and healing. The intense emotion of a man confronting his own mortality in Ingmar Bergman's classic film *Wild Strawberries* has haunted a generation. The need for healing of Willie Loman, in *Death of a Salesman*, shouts to the audience. Current ethical debate about the effect of watching violent death daily on television, and its potential contribution to increasing rates of acts of violence, is evidence of the power of the media in influencing attitudes and behaviors.

Ritual

One reason that art in its many forms is so powerful is that it often makes use of the rituals of death. Rituals of death include:

- *people*, including funeral directors, nurses and physicians, clergy, and others who are associated with the dying
- *places*, such as cemeteries, battlefields, and funeral chapels, which exist either to honor the dead or which provide a special place for rites to occur
- *special times* for remembrance of the dead, such as Veteran's Day or Memorial Day
- *special objects* associated with death, such as obituaries, hearses, and tombstones
- *special symbols*, such as skull and crossbones or a black arm band (Doyle, Hanks, & MacDonald, 1993, p. 34)

Melding these symbols of death and dying can provide a rich tapestry for art, connecting with both rational study and emotion, and rooted in the values of the people—the things they consider right or wrong. The images they portray become the patterns of behavior that are followed in life as people come to believe this is the correct way to behave. One comes to believe that suicide is wrong when a powerful poem conveys the suffering of parents following the suicide death of a teen. While desensitization to suicide may occur if the word or concept is simply repeated in a superficial way many times, desensitization does not seem to occur when art gives the term feeling and connection to self, when it becomes personal.

Rituals of death are also rooted in the culture. Cultures may view death in several ways. Some cultures are death-accepting, and others are death-denying. Some may even be termed death-defying (Kearl, 1989, p. 26). Death may be a process, or a state. Cultures may view death as an end to life, or as a transition to another form of life. If it is seen as a transition, the concept of immortality may be one of personal transition or of collective transition. Hindus believe that the life between reincarnations is the real (or objective) world, and that the current life is an illusion. Americans, on the other hand, believe what is felt, seen, and heard is real, and the notion of another world is quite illusory. Even so, the illusory world past death holds promise for another kind of life, and so funeral customs may be as much a passage to another life as a farewell to this one.

Historically, funeral and burial rites have been both symbolic and useful. They reinforce beliefs of a society about death. For example, the kings of Egypt, buried as Tutankhamen was, with food, riches, personal keepsakes, and treasures, reinforced the belief of the time that such items would be of value in the hereafter. That contrasts with modern views of Americans who believe that "you can't take it with you." An expensive coffin in the United States is more often a sign of respect for the dead than an attempt to influence what happens after burial.

Funeral rites are comforting to individuals as they realize they are part of a greater whole, a family or a clan. Rites provide a place to begin the bereavement process, to talk safely and without the discomfort that so often accompanies conversation about death, especially in a death-denying society. The rites often include a *wake*—a visitation with family and friends for mutual support and comfort. At a traditional Irish wake, family and friends remember, toast, and celebrate the deceased. Sometimes the rites provide a place and a formal time to say good-bye to the person who has died or to complete unfinished business with that person. A serviceperson, called home after the death of a parent, may look at the familiar face in the coffin and kiss it one last time, or say "thank you" for the things not recognized before, or just say "good-bye." To remember one who has been cremated, the ashes may be scattered in a place of personal meaning, leading to a release of grief. Rites are society's way of creating a structure in which a set of behaviors is taught to help members of that society deal with grief and loss, or to celebrate and memorialize group members. That structure changes slowly over time as societal values and attitudes change.

MORTALITY THROUGH THE AGES

Mr. Bower, whom we met in Chapter 1, lived in the hospital with his disease for 8 months. He could do so because of the technology and care available to treat him. He was 49 years old when he died. That is approximately the number of years he could have been expected to live if he had been born in England in 1900 (Lancaster, 1990, p. 44). For most citizens of the United States, 49 years seems young. In fact, in 1989, the life expectancy for white men born in the United States was 73 years (U.S. Bureau of the Census, 1992). A man who was 73 years old in 1989 would have lived through several periods of high mortality rates (his first year of life; his teenage years, prone to infection and/or violence; middle-age years, which predisposed him to cardiovascular disease and some cancers). Having survived those things, he could be expected to live another 10 years.

Minority groups have a somewhat shorter life expectancy than the cultural majority groups. This is most likely related to the greater proportion of minority groups living in restricted economic conditions. Inner city violence kills more minority teens than Caucasian teens, sometimes because of gang culture, and often because they happen to live in a certain area in which violence is endemic. Some diseases such as diabetes and cardiovascular disease are more deadly in groups with limited access to health care. That limited access may be due to distance from a health care setting, insufficient numbers of health care professionals in an area, or too few resources with which to purchase care. Diseases specific to cultural groups, such as Thalassemia, or diseases that affect only a few people, such as multiple sclerosis, may receive fewer research dollars, so cure may be delayed. Diseases that affect a minority group of people may require expensive treatments which few people can afford. The only known possible cure for sickle cell anemia, a disease affecting primarily African American people, is bone marrow transplant. That treatment is not only extremely expensive, but depends on finding appropriate bone marrow donors. While matches between donors and those needing bone marrow will be found most frequently in a similar racial group (because blood types are genetically determined), African Americans have a low rate of giving blood or organs for transplant. If this trend continues for bone marrow, cure for sickle cell anemia will not be widely available.

Mortality Before the Industrial Revolution

How long a person is likely to live, and how she is likely to die, is largely a function of the society and the times in which she lives. Before the industrial revolution, a typical deathbed scene involved a young mother and father desperately trying to save the feverish infant who was so young its only means of expression was to cry. Too often, the parents were unsuccessful. Nearly as likely was the deathbed scene in which the mother, having had several children already, died during childbirth. The youthful widower was left with the other children, sometimes a newborn, and often without the means to care for them all. The newborn may have died of starvation if a wet nurse could not be found, because lack of refrigeration prevented storing milk.

Mortality rates for any one region varied according to the presence or absence of epidemic, for which there was no known cure, or of famine, an equally uncontrollable event. Contagious diseases afflicted those who lived along popular highways or in dense populations, and those who had little resistance to disease. Contributing to inadequate resistance to disease was poor nutritional status, almost nonexistent hygiene (lack of running water, sewer systems), and other environmental factors.

From the Industrial Revolution to World War II

After the industrial revolution, social conditions began to change. Working conditions improved, and there were developments in agriculture, housing, sanitation, communication, and public health. People born in 1930 had a life expectancy of over 60 years. By the 1950s, life expectancy in the United States was over 70 years. With a few exceptions, most notably the development of antibiotics and widespread use of vaccines, medical developments were not credited for the extension of life expectancy. Social change was believed responsible for increasing the number of years of life. Social change is in the hands of the public, and the changes created were based on the values of the times.

Deathbed scenes after the industrial revolution moved to the older aged groups. People died at home during the first part of the twentieth century, more often of prolonged disease, such as cancer, and of infections such as tuberculosis or meningitis. They had time to call in the family to the bedside, and name their heirs, say good-bye, and give their blessings to the caregivers and loved ones. In the second half of the twentieth century, two major shifts occurred that changed the way people thought of and dealt with death.

Post World War II

During World War II, the role of women began changing rapidly. Women worked in industry during the war, and did not give up their jobs after the war. Immediately after the war, many families became dependent on the incomes of two adults or a single head of household when there was only one adult in the home. Fewer women took on the traditional role of full-time housewife and family caretaker. When family members, particularly the aged, became ill, they were hospitalized, often for extended periods of time. Eventually, it became the norm for the person who was not going to get well to complete the dying process in the hospital, though all the hospital staff could accomplish was palliative care. By tacit agreement, hospitalization was prolonged, in part so that the family could continue with their work without interruption.

Their paid sick days covered only the employee, so lost days of work meant lost pay at the time when money was needed to cover the expenses of the sick or dying family member. The longer the hospital was willing to keep the patient (covered by insurance, of course), the fewer days off the caregiver had to take. Society had not defined the appropriate place or caregiver of palliative care. Hospice was valued, but not yet widespread. Home care was viewed as difficult, and people unskilled in caregiving did not know what their roles were. In the early part of the century, private duty nurses were available and were hired by the wealthy to care for loved ones at home until they died. In the decades between 1950 and 1990, the most common model of care took place in the hospital, given or supervised by professional nurses.

The advent of prospective payment system (payment for hospitalization based on diagnosis and the average length of time a person needed hospital care for reasons related to medical and nursing care) ended the use of hospitals for extended maintenance care. But a whole generation had grown up never seeing death, except in the special death place of the funeral home. Death occurred in hospitals, out of sight.

A second reason for the change in the way people thought of death in the second half of the twentieth century was the extended and seemingly ever increasing use of technology. The Korean and Vietnam wars are often credited with the initial explosion of the use of impressive technologic developments for trauma patients. Machines were developed to take over major functions of the body, like breathing (ventilators), exchanging body waste (dialysis), or monitoring functions such as electrical impulses (electroencephalography, cardiac telemetry), or pressures (ventricular screws or Swanz-ganz catheters). Nurses, physicians, and family members often felt caught in a kind of moral dilemma. The values of the American society as a whole suggested that all human life was worth preserving, that death was to be postponed, and that there was always the chance of the miracle in which the patient would suddenly become alert and whole. The cost in terms of dignity of the patient, possible pain, and other kinds of suffering was overridden by the finality of death and the implication that everything possible was not done for the person. Family members would feel guilty if they considered financial ruin a cause for ending treatment, and health care team members felt a sense of failure when death occurred. Death deformed life; it was not a natural process.

Being present for the death of a loved one or having the dying person in the home, and believing that death should be avoided at all costs for as long as possible seems to have led many Americans to imagine a kind of *technologic death*, because they have not seen a peaceful death. A technologic death occurs when a dying person is kept alive via a variety of machines. Many people have a vision of tubes in every opening of the body dripping fluid either in or out, sensors sending information translated into beeps, the soft bubbling and whoosh of artificial breathing, and personhood suspended in some unknown state. While this view of death is often inaccurate, it is perpetuated by television and movies, often a worst case scenario. The process of death is feared, ironically, for the very lack of dignity that the available technology requires when used to prolong the end of life.

Some people would like to fight death to the end, and use every available resource to assist in the fight. They want to taste every drop of life, good or bad. Others wish to avoid the extremes and make choices based on other values, such as comfort or dignity. Legal issues regarding who has the right or the obligation to limit the use of technology to sustain life or prolong death and under what circumstances must be defined. Attempts to end the use of technology that is sustaining life can result in long delays and conflict between individuals, families, and society as represented by the law.

The legal problems encountered by people who want to limit the use of technology to extend life came about initially because of mandates intended to preserve and protect the public. Society feared that someone other than the dying individual would make an irrevocable decision to forgo life support contrary to the wishes of the person. Living wills and informed consent laws are society's attempts to give some choice about the dying process to those experiencing it. Without such choice, the modern deathbed scene usually takes place in the hospital, with the one who is dying surrounded by machines that make jarring noises and lights, and strangers who are busy with many tasks, who feel their responsibility is to fight death to the end. The wish for a peaceful death is a vague hope.

Death at Present

Without trauma due to accident or violence, people born in the United States have an even chance of living to the age of 85. Riley (1989, p. 11) called this the maximum average life span, or *modal age of death*. Some groups are at higher risk for earlier death, but researchers now agree that people probably have genetic limitations on life span, and that further prolongation of life without genetic change is unlikely. Others believe that the modal age of death will increase to a maximum achievable age of 110 in groups who make social changes toward maximum health. Even so, in the next decade the majority of deaths will occur either as technologic deaths in modern trauma centers, the result of increasing violence, suicide, and accident rates, or in old age. As political forces wrestle with health care reform issues, sites of extended care for the elderly are likely to be varied according to the social and economic status of the population. Some groups will value home care and learn the skills to care for the loved one who is dying. They will receive support from the larger society, and allow the elderly to die at home. Others will be comfortable receiving help from long-term care facilities. Family members will seek places where around-the-clock care will be provided in safe and pleasant surroundings, protecting the patient's choices and dignity. Those who wish to be present at the patient's death will be called, and new rituals will be created to meet the needs of the bereaved and the dying person. Callahan (1993) suggested that if society begins to value the idea of a peaceful death, everything that interferes with peace must be justified. This means that lights, tubes, noises, and people in the patient's environment would be limited to that which contribute to comfort. Doctors would have the responsibility of deciding when medical treatment would not serve to contribute to either cure or comfort. For example, if cardiopulmonary resuscitation (CPR) were unlikely to be successful, it would not be started, since to do so would only be an act of violence toward the dying patient (Youngner, 1988). Fighting for life at any cost would be seen as one choice of several. A peaceful death would become more common, more possible.

Political, economic, and ethical debates take place before society changes, and it is in those debates that nurses have the chance to influence how dying will occur for patients in the future. The debate takes place at all levels of society: in Congress during health care reform and in financing decisions; in think tanks like the Hastings Center for Ethics; and in the institutions devoted to education, religion, and health care. These are all social institutions, and the nurse who wishes to remain informed about healing the dying needs to monitor and perhaps contribute to the debate.

PEACEFUL DEATH: LETTING GO

Mr. Kashu

Mr. Kashu was planning to go home tomorrow. His pneumonia was almost resolved, as was seen on the chest x-ray. The antibiotics had been changed from I.V. to oral, so that he could take them at home and continue his recovery. On this day, the mail contained a letter from his married son, which he thought contained arrangements for going home. He was wrong. The short letter told him of his son's plan to divorce his wife. The son informed Mr. Kashu that the responsibility for the divorce was Mr. Kashu's, since he had not helped his son enough over the years. The son blamed the father for everything that had gone wrong in his life. After reading the letter, the middle-aged man looked up and said, "It's time to die now." He lay on his bed and let go of his life. He was pronounced dead 30 minutes later. No physical cause could be found for his death.

Euthanasia, suicide, and prolonged extension of life past one's desire to live would not be issues today if people believed that they had the skill to decide to die, and then did so. There would be no need to consider some of the most important ethical issues of our time. But there is abundant evidence that people do have such abilities. It is well-documented that in many societies individuals die without a demonstrable physical cause. Sometimes it may be related to a sadness, as with Mr. Kashu. Sometimes the physical cause can be inferred, as in the case of Eskimo elders who, in the past, chose not to be a burden on their social group by floating away from the group on an ice floe when they felt that they had outlived their usefulness. One can imagine hypothermia, drowning, or starvation to be the cause of death. Sometimes the fact that a person believes that she will die seems sufficient to bring the death about.

Many cultures have a powerful spiritual person, Shaman, or witch who has the ability to hex or cast a spell on a person, which causes sickness or death without obvious physical contact. Voodoo priestesses in New Orleans were at one time thought to mix a variety of things, including the plaster from a broken statue of a saint and dirt from a fresh grave taken at midnight, and use the resulting powder to cause harm or death to enemies.

Conversely, most nurses and physicians know a patient who came to the hospital with a severe disease and was not expected to live. Yet years later the former patient is clearly a survivor, and no one knows why; many people with far fewer symptoms and less severe disease have died. It would seem that such people possess the quality of hardiness. They have the ability to hold onto life despite many challenges. Health care providers also know people who have lived long enough to achieve a goal in spite of great odds. Sometimes they live long enough to participate in some family event, like the birth of a grandchild, marriage of a child, a wedding anniversary, or a visit from a person important to them.

There seems to be a quality about some people, a personal characteristic that allows them some internal control over letting go of life or holding on to it a bit longer. That ability is not likely to be useful in prolonging life beyond the allotted life span, but it may be useful in allowing individuals to die a peaceful death. That internal control may be conditioned by society and culture. The meaning of death in the culture may provide the individual the opportunity to accept or reject an active role in the death process.

SUMMARY

People die within society, not apart from it. Values and attitudes toward death are taught and conditioned by the society in which one lives. Social conditions like sanitation and nutrition predispose one to health or illness. Whether a group of people chooses to confront death or deny it is determined at least in part by the mores of the whole society. Language and other symbols, such as art, literature, and drama, condition people to think of death in certain ways.

Death rates have changed through the years. Although there seems to be a finite number of years of life, the greatest number of deaths in any generation has risen from the time when most people who were born died in infancy, to a time when infection and plague decimated the population, to a time when most people have a reasonable expectation of dying in old age. For most of human history, it was reasonable to fight to achieve longer life, because death was premature when compared to the standard of 85 years. Technologic death has been accepted because the technology used provided a reasonable hope of restoring the person to society. Now, however, prolongation of life as a societal goal is being reviewed, and the goal of a peaceful death reconsidered. This apparent conflict of goals has led to frequent, impassioned debate, a debate in which nurses should certainly take part.

References

Callahan, D. (1993) "Pursuing a peaceful death." *The troubled dream of life: Living with mortality* (chapter 6). New York: Simon & Schuster.

Doyle, D., Hanks, G. W. C., & MacDonald, N. (Eds.). (1993). *Oxford textbook of palliative medicine*. Oxford: Oxford University Press.

Hamilton, D. (1991). Vital energy: the antebellum health movement. *Journal of Holistic Nursing, 9*(3), 10–19.

Kearl, M. C. (1989). *Endings: A sociology of death and dying*. New York: Oxford University Press.

Lancaster, H. O. (1990). *Expectations of life: A study in the demography, statistics, and history of world mortality*. New York: Springer-Verlag.

Riley, J. C. (1989). *Sickness, recovery and death: A history and forecast of ill health.* Iowa City, Iowa: University of Iowa Press.

U.S. Bureau of the Census. Statistical Abstracts of the U.S.: 1992 (Ed. 112). Washington, DC, p. 76.

Youngner, S. J. (1988). Who defines futility? *Journal of the American Medical Association, 260,* 2094–2095.

3 THEORIES RELATED TO DYING, HEALING

THE USEFULNESS OF THEORY

Nursing practice is guided by theory. Relevant theory provides a framework that suggests to the practitioner what has happened, what to look for, how to measure an event, and what treatments or actions are most likely to yield some desirable outcome. Theories are not mutually exclusive. They may be used together if they use common terminology and concepts.

Theories are not always identified as theories. They are taught as a way of doing things, and they become patterns of behavior. An example is the nursing process. It is taught to almost all nursing students as a way of providing nursing care for all patients. Nurses learn to assess, plan, treat, and evaluate care. It becomes a standard, a pattern of behavior that nurses share in caring for patients.

Nursing theories are attempts by nurses to look at the theoretical foundations of the discipline of nursing. They may be based on even larger theory, such as general systems theory from science or phenomenological theory from philosophy. Nursing theories are broad and can accommodate the addition of mid-range theories. Mid-range theories help focus on smaller areas of interest in the care of patients. They can be useful in further developing the way nurses address the care of grieving, dying patients and their families.

Different theorists have studied concepts and relationships of grief, families, and self-transcendence. Grief theory aims to describe the grief process and to develop useful ways to help people resolve grief. It describes the significance of resolution of grief in people's lives. Combining family theory and grief theory is useful in helping the family members to resolve grief in order to help the dying person while living their own lives. Self-transcendence as a theory focuses on an inner connectedness that helps move people toward peace and meaning in life.

GRIEF THEORY

Grief is a universal human experience. It is also intensely personal. Understanding what is universal and allowing the expression of what is personal help the nurse to plan sensitive, effective care for dying people and their families.

Definitions

Sometimes the term *grief* is used synonymously with loss, mourning, or bereavement. There are subtle differences (see table 3.1). Grief is the internal sadness resulting from loss, and cannot be measured in time. Loss (of someone or something meaningful) precipitates the states of bereavement and mourn-

Term	Definition
Loss:	absence of someone or something meaningful.
Bereavement:	a response to the loss of something, or someone.
Mourning:	a feeling or expression of sorrow or sadness following loss.
Depression:	1) sadness gone awry. 2) A clinical diagnosis of an illness which sometimes follows significant loss. It can be treated successfully in most people. 3) A stage of grief in some theories, which is normal if not prolonged.

TABLE 3.1   *Definitions of Terms Related to Grief*

ing. Mourning is a connection with cultural rituals, acting out feelings of sadness. In some cultures, a young widow who is in mourning may wear black for a year following the death of her husband. The term *a period of mourning* may mean a variable period of time, perhaps a few months or a year, depending on the closeness of the bereaved to the one who died. Bereavement refers to a specific kind of loss, the death of a significant person in one's life.

Grief, as a theory, links concepts into a whole fabric of ideas that help decide action. Grief theory has its origins in psychoanalytic theory (Freud, 1957); psychology (Caplan, 1974); pastoral care (Kushner, 1981); and medicine (Lindemann, 1944; Kübler-Ross, 1969). Grief studies by nurses became more common after the publication and popularization of the works of Kübler-Ross (who is not a nurse) on the stages of grief in the 1960s. Quint (1966) was one of the first nurses to study grief systematically. Both Quint and Kübler-Ross focused on grief associated with the loss of a loved one, not on grief related to loss of goods, health, or other things.

Developmental Theory

Developmental theory classifies life into stages. Erickson's (1963) eight stages of life are well known for describing the tasks each individual should achieve before moving to the next stage, an ordered progression through life. Lindemann (1944) proposed the idea that grieving people enter a series of stages. Lindemann's stages represented five classes of symptoms that normal grieving people develop. Symptoms include somatic distress, preoccupation with the image of the deceased, guilt, hostility, and "loss of patterns of conduct" (a kind of restlessness and inability to concentrate). Lindemann's work is now considered a classic, though grief theory has developed in other directions.

The same idea of developmental stages was used by Kübler-Ross (1975) in her book *Death: The Final Stage of Growth*. Death is perceived as something to be achieved, another rung on a ladder. Such a theory allows one to contem-

	Stages 1		Through		5
Kübler-Ross: Coping with Dying	Denial	Anger	Bargaining	~~Depression~~	Acceptance
Bowlby	Protest	Despair		Detachment	Resolution

TABLE 3.2   Comparison of Stages of Grief

plate a variety of philosophies relating to what happens after death. Kübler-Ross identified five stages that grieving people normally use to cope with their losses. Much earlier, Bowlby (1961) had noted four different stages of grieving. Their respective stages are compared in table 3.2.

Developmental theorists point out that the stages they identify are not mutually exclusive. A grieving person may go back and forth between them, often quite quickly. A grieving person may be denying the death of a loved one, but in only a few minutes become very angry about it. Or a person may begin to regain control, only to slip back into withdrawal on a subsequent day. Stages of grief are transient.

Characteristics of Grief

Cowles and Rodgers (1991) analyzed the nursing and medical literature to define grief. They defined grief as "a pervasive, highly individualized, dynamic process that often is discussed normatively within professional disciplines."

Grief is pervasive. It has the potential to affect every aspect of life. One can develop physical symptoms, such as inability to swallow, feeling of palpitations in the heart, hyperventilation, and others, as a response to grief. It can be hard to make decisions or to do the things one usually does. Thoughts, behaviors, and feelings are all affected. One tends to be preoccupied with the one who died (or is dying), cannot concentrate on what others may be saying, does not want to make choices, or makes choices without much thought. This intense kind of grief is termed *acute*, though it can recur long after the death.

Grief is also individualized. How people respond to grief depends on:

- the nature of their relationship with the one lost
- presence of a support system
- previous losses in their lives
- religious background
- cultural beliefs about how to grieve

No one grieves quite like anyone else and no one resolves grief like anyone else. The ability to use grief to reach a new level of experience is also variable.

Grief is dynamic. Cowles and Rodgers (1991) used the word *dynamic* to indicate the changing, moving nature of grief. They found little evidence of phases, but of feelings, thought, and sensations flowing back and forth. Grief seems to be viewed more as a process, as work to be done, as clusters of activity. Bowlby (1961) visualized a spiral figure that illustrated the progress of grief through life, in which each grief experience passed through the same behaviors and feelings as the previous grief experience. While earlier theorists suggest a time period of six months to two years to move through the grief process, many now find that it may be limitless. Anniversaries of special times, including the loss itself, or special days like Memorial Day, may rekindle the emotions and revive grief (Hess, 1990).

Grief is normative. That is, grief is defined by society and culture to be normal, or atypical, or pathological. The way a person responds to grief is given a value judgment by the group one lives with, according to the group's norms. This is particularly true in the professional disciplines. The hospital is a particular kind of environment. Immediately after the death of a loved one, family or friends are expected to make decisions about organ donation, or choice of funeral home, or whom to call first. If they cry, staff may be uncomfortable, but if they don't, they may risk being seen as cold or unfeeling.

Consequences of Grief

People going through the dynamic process of grief in their own ways, but tied to their society by cultural mores, achieve two long-term consequences. They seem to develop a new reality and a new sense of self (identity). The new reality is that for the families there are new roles that do not include the deceased. There may also be new circumstances for the survivors, such as changed financial status or feeling less welcome at events for couples only. These new roles, which are forced on the survivors, cause survivors to think and act differently. In order to take on new roles, family members may need to learn to do new things, like managing finances. A new widow may learn to play bridge as a way to meet people. Inevitably, these changes force a change in how people think about themselves.

A bereaved person has choices. The new identity might include pride in accomplishing tasks or refusal to consider necessary change, which will lead to continued sadness and continued grieving. In American society, grieving too long is called *dysfunctional grieving*, thereby giving it the connotation of illness. The rationale for that is the inability to function appropriately in society. The consequences of grief for the dying person include the new reality and the new identity, but there is less time to achieve these things, and less energy. Hess (1990) described three clinical phases that occur between the time the dying person recognizes that death is imminent, and death itself. They are: (1) acute crisis; (2) chronic living-dying; and (3) terminal. These phases are pervasive, individual, and dynamic, as grief is for those who are not dying. They give some structure for caregivers to assist the dying individual with achievement of the tasks of dying.

In all phases, there should be a focus on creating an environment that is accepting of individual differences, supports the dying person in creating appropriate relationships with family and friends, and gives as much control over the living-dying process as the dying person is willing to take. The acute phase, in which the person and family and friends have learned of a fatal diagnosis, is an unstable period. Crisis intervention is commonly needed to help them refocus, deal with small losses as they occur, and support the cycle of denial and hope, which allows them to continue in a meaningful relationship for the time remaining.

Often, the chronic living-dying stage will continue for some time. The person who is dying must integrate care (e.g., chemotherapy, regular stress-tests, and so on) into an already full program of work, family, and social obligations. A priority must be placed on doing those things that are important to accomplish in the life span remaining, and to conserve energy and time. Decisions to take an active role in treatment, including the less traditional activities of massage, imagery, and meditation, should be advocated to the extent that they support hope and move a person toward hardiness. Continued evaluation and changes in the schedule of things to be done takes into account diminishing energy and ability. The same planning should be done to accomplish the resolution of psychological tasks and things the person wants to do before death. Family members often ask what they should do. It is important for them to understand that at times, the best thing to do is to *be*. Being requires the ability to sit quietly, perhaps hold hands or touch, and just share the same room. That may be what is needed at that moment. Relationships should be a priority. The ability to resolve an old argument with a parent, to leave a message for children, or to say goodbye in a meaningful way to a spouse allows the person to work toward a sense that life has had meaning.

The terminal phase finds the person drawing inward. Most tasks have been accomplished or abandoned. More physical support is required during this time, as well as time to be quiet. Friends and family may talk quietly, but not require much interaction with the dying one. Hope changes from a wish for remission or miracle cures to comfort with what is, an integration or acceptance of impending death.

FAMILY THEORY

Like grief theory, family theory provides guidance for nursing practice. There are two reasons for that. Everyone is a product of a family and an emotional system. Each individual is a part of a greater whole. Mr. Bower (chapter 1) initially said he had no family. But he was a veteran and his compatriots were very much like his family. When any one of them died, all of them grieved. The dying person grieves with family, and when death comes, the family left behind continues to grieve. The family often needs nursing support.

The second reason family theory is important in the study of dying is that families provide the support for a dying member. Families have the potential for helping the dying person, or making the dying more difficult. So it is an important part of the nursing role to assess the potential for support by family, and the need they may have for intervention.

Types of Families

There are many types of families. Three family types have traditionally been identified. The family of origin is the one a person is born into (or enters into at a very early age), and includes mother, father, brothers, and sisters. This group is also the nuclear family for the parents. The nuclear family is the family of "marriage, parenthood, or procreation" (Friedman, 1986). It includes mother, father, and their children. The extended family includes those relationships by blood or marriage in the next level from the nuclear family. They are grandparents, aunts and uncles, and cousins.

There are many people who do not live in any of those types of families. Friedman (1986) defined family as "two or more people who are emotionally involved with each other and live in close geographical proximity." Using that definition, several other family types can be identified. Family forms include:

- single parent family
- kin network (living alone, near relatives)
- cohabitating couple
- commune
- homosexual union

The word *family*, when linked with other words, may give more definition to these structures. For example, the adoptive family may be a nuclear family, with one or more of the children having been adopted.

Family Theories

Like grief theory, family theory has its origins in psychoanalytic theory, psychology, sociology, and related disciplines. The Becvars (1988) began a history of family therapy in the 1930s and 1940s, citing such diverse contributors to the interdisciplinary approach as cybernetics and anthropology.

Family theory may be categorized as either a developmental theory or a systems theory, depending on the theorist. Interaction theory and structural/functional theory are also useful frameworks (see table 3.3). The unit of analysis, or the focus of the theory, is the whole family. Individuals make up the family, and so are of interest in terms of how they relate within the family.

Approach	Focus
Development	Family is a small group, progressing through identified stages over a life cycle.
Interactional	Family is a set of interacting personalities.
Structural/functional	Family is a social system that has characteristics of a small group and functions that serve both individual family members and society.
Systems	Family is an open social system that uses feedback for self-regulation, and individuals are subsystems that interact within the family and beyond the family.

TABLE 3.3   Approaches to Family Theory

Developmental Family Theory

Developmental family theory views the family as having a life cycle. There are tasks the family does at different points in the cycle. Duvall (1977) formulated eight "core developmental tasks," which paralleled his family life cycle. The family begins with a marriage, expands through childbearing, preschool, school-age, teenagers, and launching. It then begins to contract through stages of middle-age and aging. The role of each individual in the family is designed to achieve the tasks of the group. Family tasks include:

- provision of shelter and necessities, including health care
- allocation of resources
- determination of individual tasks (who does what)
- socialization
- establishment of ways of interacting
- child rearing
- community life
- developing family loyalties and values

The way in which family members react to grief is determined to a large extent by how each accomplishes the identified tasks. What they believe about health, how they socialize with each other, the extended family, and other people, and their values all give direction to their relationship with the person dying (or with themselves, if they are dying). Using a developmental framework in which to plan care for a grieving family, the nurse would assess which stage of development the family is in, knowing that grief is different at different stages in the family's life. A child's death would signal unfulfilled potential, unfinished tasks, while death of the aged may be fulfillment of expectation. Affection may be available to some but not to other family members. Certain behaviors, like withdrawal, may be unacceptable in some, depending on their expected role. An eldest son may be expected to deliver the eulogy at his father's funeral, while his mother is free to cry.

When Duvall began his theory development, families were less complex, and generally thought of as nuclear families. While Duvall's theory was a beginning, the changing nature of the American family meant that theorists began looking at families in different ways. Many tasks of families that Duvall identified continue to be relevant. For example, socialization, the provision of shelter, and the establishment of consistent values occur within the family structure, no matter what form a particular family may take. But child rearing for a childless couple or differentiation of tasks in a single adult home is only meaningful as it relates to the larger family, and family theories are moving away from developmental theories to other models. It is probably more efficient to view families in a different way than to try to trace the developmental stages for each of the forms of family that now exist.

Structural/Functional Family Theory

Friedman (1986) attempted to integrate family structure and function to create a useful model of family care. She identified four structural dimensions of family:

- role structure
- value systems
- communication processes
- power structure

Using the idea of outcomes of family structure as functions, she integrated five functions of families (affective function, or personality maintenance for individuals; socialization, primarily of the children; reproduction; economic function; and health care function). Each member of the family has a defined role and position. The role may be functional, such as the person who kisses the hurt and makes it well, or it may be based on position, for example, parent.

When the loss of a family member is anticipated, the role of the dying person must be reassigned, and tasks redistributed. If this is done before the death occurs, the person dying may feel left out, devalued. Or the dying one may share in decisions and develop a feeling of continuity with the family even if absent. If the role is left unfilled, the family may suffer. Working out the new ways each family member must relate to other family members with sensitivity and compassion is a task of the family. They may require help in knowing when the dying family member is ready to give up the role or to accept help with it.

Family Systems Theory

Systems theory views families as social systems that are self-regulating. They identify their own boundaries by identifying those who are included in the family or with whom the family chooses to interact. Individuals are components of the system. Specific pathways of communication are required to maintain family health. Disruption such as grief requires new channels of communication and affords the opportunity to create new ways of relating.

Two major concepts of family systems theory are feedback (communication) and adaptation. An open family (one that welcomes new ideas, actively problem solves, and interacts with the larger community) generally has established communication systems within the family and with the community. This gives access to support systems, means of expressing feelings, and outlets for emotions that are acceptable to the family. By contrast, a closed family is distrustful, controlling its members by force, and focused on predictability in relationships. Communication is by standard, proscribed means. A family that is too open does not filter or evaluate the information it receives, and can become disorganized and chaotic. A family that is too closed does not receive enough information and cannot change.

Adaptation is seen as cyclical. The family strives for stability, for maintaining preferred patterns of behavior as long as possible because it helps to develop a feeling of security. But demands of the community and home environment occur, requiring change. For example, an adolescent begins to date. Perhaps the zoning laws change and the neighbors start to raise chickens. Or a loved one is diagnosed with an incurable disease. How the family responds to each of these events, how it adapts, depends on how it evaluates the information in terms of family values and goals, and patterns of communication and behavior it has developed over time.

Family systems theory has been developed into several specific forms of family therapy, all building upon the principles of systems. Three of the more useful theorists for nursing care are Virginia Satir, Salvador Minuchin, and Murray Bowen.

Grief and Family

Using the systems perspective, Walsh and McGoldrick (1991) identified two major tasks of people who are grieving. The first is "shared acknowledgment of the reality of death and shared experience of loss." The acknowledgment of death in a death-denying culture can pose real problems. If clear communication patterns have not been established within the family, and especially with the one who is dying, it may be difficult for the dying person to talk about death, to use the knowledge to finish his business and work toward a peaceful death. The family, too, may fail to use the time before the death occurs to prepare for the impending changes or say appropriate good-byes. Worse, according to Bowen (1976), they may become "stuck" in a pattern, unable to grow into new relationships after the death, reliving the death unknowingly at inappropriate times. For example, a parent who lost her mother at the age of 16, two years after she started dating, may treat her own daughter of 16 years the same way for several years in spite of the fact that her child is getting older and society expects change.

Family communication patterns may be functional or dysfunctional, and a careful assessment by the nurse to learn how information is shared in the family will help determine the need for nursing support. Bowen (1976) said that patterns in families persist for three to five generations. If some family members dominate communication patterns over two or three generations, establishing or changing patterns of communication after those persons die may require therapy for those who are left. Professionals in advanced practice nursing who specialize in communication patterns, grief work, or psychiatric nursing can help family members learn new ways to relate.

An interesting way of assessing patterns across generations is the use of genograms (see figure 3.1). Genograms are pictorial representations of family relationships, and three to five generations can be included on one form. Patterns of relationships, including how people died and at what age, major diseases, marital status of family members, including divorce, separation, singleness, and long-term marriage, are seen at a glance

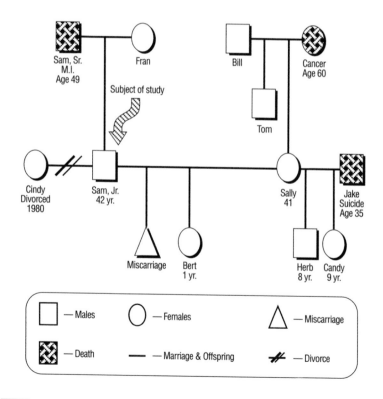

FIGURE 3.1 *Three generational genogram*

(McGoldrick & Gerson, 1985). Creating the genogram can be done with the dying person, with the family, or with both, and can help to begin a discussion about death and what it means to the family. Figure 3.1 shows Sam, Jr. as the central person of interest. His father is dead, mother living. He is divorced from his first wife. His present wife had a previous marriage and was widowed. She had two children from that marriage who are now eight and nine years old. She and Sam, Jr. married and had a child. One other pregnancy ended in miscarriage. From the genogram, it is possible to detect other family information, like whether Sally's parents are alive, and the sex of Sam's children. Genograms are efficient ways of communicating a large amount of family information.

The second major task of grieving is "reorganization of the family system and reinvestment in other relationships and life pursuits" (Walsh and McGoldrick, 1991). Sometimes women who say they want to carry on the way their deceased spouse would want are not reorganizing or investing in new relationships. On the other hand, there is Mrs. J.

Mrs. J.

Mr. J. died in July. Mrs. J's mother died in August. Both of them had experienced long illnesses, during which Mrs. J. cared for them. She had grieved a lot. In September, Mrs. J. entered the hospital for an elective coronary artery bypass operation. The nurse knew that after the death of a spouse, some surviving spouses become depressed and even die. She asked Mrs. J. why she had made the decision to have the operation at this time. Mrs. J. replied that she had loved her husband very much. During the year she had cared for both him and her mother, she had developed cardiac symptoms, including angina pectoris. She, too, knew that it looked as if she might have a death wish following the deaths of her loved ones. After discussing it with her daughter, she had decided that her appropriate course of action was to get herself in the best possible physical condition so that she could get on with her life. This meant having surgery. She planned to learn to play bridge so that she could join a bridge club and meet people. And she wanted to enjoy her grandchildren. She was reinvesting in relationships, reorganizing her life. It was interesting to note that Mrs. J's mother had lost her husband at about the same age. She had joined the senior citizens' organization, gone on regular outings with others in the church group, and had become quite active in a social way for the rest of her life. Twelve years after the surgery, Mrs. J. is 82 years old and has a steady male friend with whom she enjoys travel, concerts, and parties.

Mrs. J. is an example of successful resolution of grief. She remembers her spouse on anniversaries, but has new relationships and new patterns of living. Her life has meaning to her. She is at peace. She believes that when it is her time to die, her life will have mattered.

SELF-TRANSCENDENCE

Theories of self-transcendence are based on the assumption that a sense of connectedness between the innermost sense of self and the environment is a universal human characteristic. Self-transcendence is

> an expansion of one's conceptual boundaries inwardly through introspective activities, outwardly through concerns about others' welfare, and temporally by integrating perceptions of one's past and future to enhance the present (Reed, 1991a).

This expansion of self-boundaries orients one to a broadened sense of purpose in life. It defines meaning in life.

Self-transcendence has been studied largely in association with end-of-life issues. At the end of life, concern about meaning is a recurrent theme, and many people confronting death ask questions starting with *why* for this reason. Frankl (1963) studied concentration camp survivors to discover why some people who seemed weak survived when others, who seemed much stronger, did not. He found that those who survived found purpose and meaning even in the camp situation. For Frankl, one transcends either toward other people or toward meaning. One does so in one of three ways. It may be by creativity (either in family or in creative works). It may be by receptivity to others and the environment. Or it may be by developing an attitude of acceptance when a situation cannot be changed (Coward, 1991). Vaughn (1985) presented the following words to describe the self-transcendent person: compassionate, wise, receptive, creative, open, connected, intuitive, and spiritual. The person has moved beyond self-concern without devaluing self. Reaching out to others, the self-transcendent person develops a greater sense of meaning and purpose by helping others. Many peer support groups are led by people who find meaning in helping others cope with the same diagnoses and treatments they have had.

Self-transcendence has been linked with less depression, self-neglect, and feelings of hopelessness (Reed, 1991b). Self-transcendent people have a greater sense of well-being and the ability to cope with grief (Coward, 1991). Part of the coping ability is related to the willingness of self-transcendent people to accept and to give support. Part of it also has to do with the ability of the self-transcendent person to live in the present rather than in the past. A self-transcendent person may see death as a natural part of life.

It is unrealistic to expect all dying patients to achieve self-transcendence. Yet all people approaching the end of life should be encouraged to search for meaning or connectedness. Finding meaning and connecting with others makes grieving easier. One learns to turn an experience that is potentially devastating into a reason for hope. Sometimes transcendence occurs in a particularly short period (the *transcendent moment*), and great and lasting joy may be a component of the experience. This is often true of the person who achieves transcendence as a spiritual experience. Certainly the self-transcendent person achieves peace.

Measures to help people achieve self-transcendence build on the need to look inward, the need to connect (with family as well as others), and the need for a sense of timelessness. Life review, for example, helps a person to look at life, see that it was unique and meaningful, remember those who are loved, and realize that a place in history is reserved. Nursing measures to promote self-transcendence are included in chapter 7.

Mr. Bower, Luke, and the Nurse

Mr. Bower, a patient known for his rather stern manner, occupied a room across the hall from another patient, Luke. Luke was dying. He needed oxygen to breathe more easily, but oxygen was available in the rooms on the other side of the hallway, not in his room. Getting tanks of oxygen took time. Although it was 3 A.M., Mr. Bower saw the activity and preparations and asked what was happening. He offered to change rooms so that Luke could have the oxygen immediately. The change was made. After all the interventions that could be given had been given, Luke died at 7 A.M. Through all the frantic activity, Mr. Bower sat quietly by Luke's side. The nurse had to do the many tasks of caring for the dead that hospitals prescribe, so she was very late getting off duty. Mr. Bower walked the nurse to the elevator although he was in some pain. As she thanked him for his willingness to give up his room for the comfort of another, he said, "I sure hope you are there when it is my turn to go. You give a guy a fighting chance!" This gruff man had recognized the nurse's need for support and connected with her by acknowledging her competence and willingness to help.

SUMMARY

Theories of grief, families, and transcendence provide direction for nursing care of the dying and their families. Knowing what patterns of behavior to expect of the dying patient and family members, and the patterns the family uses for coping and relating to each other help the nurse to assess needs and determine strategies to meet those needs. Self-transcendence is a sense of connecting inwardly to the deepest sense of self and outwardly in the form of relationships with others. Achieving self-transcendence toward the end of life helps a person see that life has meaning. The realization of meaning in life helps one to live each moment fully, capable of joy and peace in spite of impending death.

References

Becvar, D. S., & Becvar, R. J. (1988). *Family therapy: A systemic integration.* Boston: Allyn and Bacon, Inc.

Bowen, M. (1976). Family reaction to death. In P. Guerin (Ed.), *Family therapy.* New York: Gardner.

Bowlby, J. (1961). Process of mourning. *International Journal of Psychoanalysis, 42,* 317.

Caplan, G. (1974). Foreward. In I. Glick, R. Weiss, & C. Parkes (Eds.), *The first year of bereavement* (pp. vi–xi). New York: Wiley.

Coward, D. (1991). Self-transcendence and emotional well-being in women with advanced breast cancer. *Oncology Nursing Forum, 18*(5), 857–863.

Cowles, K. V., & Rodgers, B. L. (1991). The concept of grief: a foundation for nursing research and practice. *Research in Nursing and Health, 14,* 119–127.

Duvall, E. M. (1977). *Marriage and family development.* Philadelphia: Lippincott.

Erickson, E. (1963). *Childhood and society.* New York: W.W. Norton & Co., Inc.

Frankl, V. (1963, ©1959). *Man's search for meaning* (3rd ed.). New York: Simon & Schuster.

Freud, S. (1957). Mourning and melancholia. In J. Strachey (Ed. and Trans.), *The standard edition of the complete psychological works of Sigmund Freud* (vol. 14, pp. 243–258). London: Hogarth Press.

Friedman, M. M. (1986). *Family nursing: Theory and assessment* (2nd ed.). Norwalk, CT: Appleton-Century-Crofts.

Hess, P. (1990). Loss, grief and dying. In P. Beare & J. L. Myers (Eds.), *Principles and practice of adult health nursing.* St. Louis: C.V. Mosby, Co.

Kübler-Ross, E. (1969). *On death and dying.* New York: Macmillan.

Kübler-Ross, E. (1975). *Death: The final stage of growth.* Englewood Cliffs, NJ: Prentiss-Hall.

Kushner, H. S. (1981). *When bad things happen to good people.* New York: Schocken Books.

Lindemann, E. (1944). Symptomatology and management of acute grief. *American Journal of Psychiatry, 101,* 141–148.

McGoldrick, M., & Gerson, R. (1985). *Genograms in family assessment.* New York: W.W. Norton & Co.

Quint, J. (1966). Awareness of death and the nurse's composure. *Nursing Research, 15,* 49–55.

Reed, P. (1991a). Self-transcendence and mental health in oldest-old adults. *Nursing Research, 40*(1), 5–11.

Reed, P. (1991b). Toward a nursing theory of self-transcendence: Deductive reformulation using developmental theories. *Advances in Nursing Science, 33*(4), 64–77.

Vaughn, F. (1985). Discovering transpersonal identity. *Journal of Humanistic Psychology, 25*(3), 13–38.

Walsh, F., & McGoldrick, M. (1991). *Living beyond loss: Death in the family.* New York: W.W. Norton & Co.

2 | COMFORT OF THE DYING INDIVIDUAL

GOALS FOR
COMFORT
IN DYING

COMFORT DEFINED

Palliative care requires that caregivers strive to help the dying person to be comfortable, even in the dying process. To strive for comfort is more than to strive to relieve pain. The goal of providing comfort and reducing discomfort for the dying person is to enable that person to live fully and satisfyingly until death occurs.

Discomfort comes from many sources. The inability to sleep, difficulty in movement, shattered dreams, and changing family roles and relationships are among the many sources of discomfort. Each of these discomforts affects the quality of a person's life.

Comfort is a multidimensional concept, meaning different things to different people. Comfort is positive and is experienced right now. It is a whole person attribute, meaning that the absence of comfort in one part of a person's existence causes the whole individual to be uncomfortable. It is not just a portion of the body, the emotions, or the spirit that suffers.

Kolcaba (1991, 1992) based her definition of comfort on patient needs. The intensity of comfort needs can be thought of as a continuum, ranging from relief on one end, through ease, and to transcendence on the other end. When a need is met, the person experiences relief. Ease occurs if the need is met and the person feels a sense of calm or serenity as a result. Transcendence occurs when the person is able to rise above negative circumstances like pain and achieve a sense of quality in life or meaning in being alive, in spite of problems. This idea of the transcendence, like the definition in chapter 3, requires the individual to reach inside himself and see the connection of self to something beyond self. Kolcaba defines comfort as "the immediate experience of having met basic human needs for relief, ease, and transcendence."

There are four kinds of internal or external comfort needs. They are

1. physical needs, or bodily sensations

2. psychospiritual, a dimension that includes awareness of self and a sense of meaning in life

3. environment, the context in which a person lives, including light, noise, odor, temperature

4. social, referring to relationships (Kolcaba, 1992)

Meeting basic human needs for comfort in the dying patient may include care within any of these four areas or any combination of them. Eliminating a noxious odor or providing a blanket changes the environment, and may provide relief or move a person into a state of ease, a higher level of comfort.

The provision of comfort has been a nursing tradition and value since Nightingale. Obviously, comfort is more than an absence of pain or absence of discomfort. Relief, as defined above, is closely related to absence of pain or discomfort, but achievement of a feeling of ease and transcendence requires that the nurse's role include those measures that improve the patient's sense of well-being and quality of life. When setting goals for patient care, it is useful to consider both comfort and quality of life as indicators of the effectiveness of care.

QUALITY OF LIFE

Quality of life has been defined as psychological, physical, social/interpersonal, and financial/material well-being (Padilla et al., 1992). Table 4.1 illustrates how closely Kolcaba's degrees of comfort needs and Padilla's components of quality of life agree. Quality of life is clearly affected by a person's level of comfort.

Comfort*	Quality of Life**
Physical	Physical
Psychospiritual	Psychological
Environment	Financial/material
Social	Social/interpersonal

TABLE 4.1   Comfort and Quality of Life

*Kolcaba
**Padilla et al.

While these theorists describe areas of life that must be considered when assisting patients to achieve a sense of well-being, others suggest that it is more complicated to decide what quality of life means. One view is that there is a gap between patient expectations of life and the reality of the situation. For example, the athlete with multiple sclerosis may expect to compete again, but the physical situation prohibits the same kind of competition as before. Quality of life in this scenario may depend on the size of the gap between the patient's expectation and the reality (Calman, 1984). The smaller the gap between expectation and reality, the greater the quality of life.

Building on that idea, a second view considers the possibility of reorganizing the strengths of an individual to achieve a new balance of mind and body, allowing a person to function at a new level. The individual achieves a different but acceptable way of living. Thus, she learns to cope with the loss of vital capacity of the lungs by walking more slowly or going out less frequently. Quality of life depends upon a person's ability to reorganize goals and abilities so that they balance.

Another view is based on the idea of a trade-off: probable length of life versus personal loss of some specific function. In one study, firefighters were more likely to choose to undergo a laryngectomy, which they were told would mean longer life, but without a voice, than businesspeople. The businesspeople felt the quality of life without a voice was unacceptable (McNeil et al., 1981). This illustrates how individual the idea of quality of life is. Comfortable, satisfying living for anyone, including the dying patient, must be evaluated by that person.

One longtime AIDS survivor credits his survival to having the financial resources to manage his environment. In addition to working with his traditional health care team, with whom he has an excellent relationship, he is able to create a peaceful, beautiful space in his backyard, growing roses and other flowers for color and enjoyment. He discusses alternative medical treatment with a variety of people he trusts, including his nurses. He chooses to stay out of crowds, limiting his risk of contracting contagious diseases. He regularly plans and gets comfort treatments, which he identifies as massage, Therapeutic Touch, and herbal treatments. His physician is fully aware of his self-medication with herbs and other over-the-counter medications, and supports his choices. He has many friends. It has been more than eight years since his first fevers were diagnosed as AIDS. His T-lymphocyte levels and other measures of potential decline have not changed, though he has had bouts of recurrent fevers and splenomegaly, requiring a splenectomy. He focuses on living a life in which he can be comfortable in each area of his life. It is his full-time job. His retirement income makes much of that possible.

This survivor is an example of a person using resources to live well. While not all patients have such resources, most have some choices to make about their environment. Assessment of the patient's ability to identify and create an appropriate environment in which living well is possible is a part of the nursing assessment.

ASSESSMENT

Assessment helps to identify problems and makes it possible to plan to address them. Spending time doing an assessment has the added benefit of establishing trust between the health care provider and the patient. Areas of quality of life that are important to assess in people who are ill include physical function, emotional or spiritual function, social function, and symptoms of disease or side effects of treatment (Doyle et al., 1993) (see table 4.2). It is important to get a list of all the doctors involved in care and to know who is coordinating care. There are also specific forms to be used to assess individual problems, such as pain or mobility, which are discussed later.

A complete history of the illness
  Chronological history of illness development
  History of treatments accepted
  Present symptoms
  Methods the patient uses to control them
Physical examination
Social history
  Occupation
  Family history
  Conditions at home
  Caregivers
  Social groups
  Participation in religious organizations
Functional assessment

TABLE 4.2   Assessment Components

Functional assessment helps identify how well a person is coping with and living in a personal environment. Discomfort of any kind limits a person's abilities to control a setting, to achieve a set of aims, or to enjoy life. The individual making treatment decisions will make those decisions based on expected ability to function, ability to rebalance her strengths, satisfaction with the course of action, and available resources.

One of the earliest and still most comprehensive guides available for functional assessment was developed for the assessment of the elderly. The OARS Multidimensional Functional Assessment Questionnaire, developed at Duke University, is divided into two sections, the first related to individual functioning, and the second identifying the utilization of services. Each section takes about 35 minutes to complete.

Table 4.3 lists the topics covered in the OARS guide. This kind of form is useful because it is comprehensive, has been widely published (so is available), and gives enough information about what a person needs to be helpful in planning care. Based on the information, a nurse can determine which areas require further assessment. For example, a patient with a history of frequent falls may need to have his home assessed for hazards such as loose rugs, lack of support rails or bars in the bathroom, or

Personal:	
Mental status	Living situation
Relationships	Economic resources
Physical health	Mobility
Sleep patterns	Activities of daily living

Services:	
Transportation	Social/recreational services
Employment services	Educational services
Supervision	Placement services
Housekeeper services	Meal preparation
Legal, protective	Overall evaluation

Care required, by category:

Nursing

Pharmacy

Physical therapy

Psychiatric

TABLE 4.3   Topics in OARS Functional Assessment

Source: Duke University Center for the Study of Aging, 1975.

dark areas of the house. These things become a problem for the patient at home who has medications that cause changes in sensorium and balance, or who has mobility problems and needs to hold on to handrails. Families may think of these things as elders become more frail, but they may not think of them when younger family members are sick and become frail. A major reason for doing a complete functional assessment is to prevent problems that interfere with maintaining the highest quality of life possible for as long as possible for the person who is dying.

Functional and hazards assessments are repeated as the patient's condition changes. Increasing frailty, dementia and confusion, and discomfort may require changes in care. For example, a patient who uses public transportation to visit the doctor's office may be required to step 18 inches up from the ground to the bus step. If that becomes impossible, other transportation arrangements may need to be made for doctor's visits. Changed plans might include being driven by family or friends, having home nursing services so that fewer visits are required to the doctor's office, or beginning to investigate hospice services or long-term care facilities for placement. Functional assessments that are used to plan ahead relieve the fear and the concern patient and family have when the situation requires change. Transition has been thought out, resources brought to the problem, and crisis avoided.

COMFORT FOR THE WHOLE PERSON

There are several ways of caring for individuals that help them deal with discomfort. They include the use of presence, surveillance and safety, providing choice, and care of the environment.

Presence

The concept of presence is a prerequisite to providing comfort that leads to the achievement of an improved quality of life. Hines (1987, p. 18) defined presence as "a mode of being available in a situation with the wholeness of one's unique individual being; a process resulting in an exchange of authentic meaningful awareness and essence linking and . . . ultimate realization of human potential." When two people are in a healing relationship, the aim is to produce a feeling of well-being, comfort, and growth. The nurse often shares this feeling with the patient. The patient usually is better able to cope as a result of the general feeling of comfort.

Characteristics of a relationship in which there is presence include: spending some time together; a nonjudgmental relationship; verbal and nonverbal communication and caring; identification of the encounter as meaningful; connectedness—being open and honest in the relationship; and something Hines terms *sustaining memory*. Sustaining memory "involves presence in absence and the memorable impression and enduring impact made between individuals in the situation that affords comfort" (Hines, 1992; Pettigrew, 1988). For the dying person, this may be the recognition that "my life matters to this nurse." Mr. Bower's nurse has a sustaining memory of him, and he knew that he would be remembered after his death.

When two people connect in a healing relationship, the patient feels that she has been heard. That is, the nurse or caregiver recognizes what the patient is saying, and trusts that the patient has knowledge of changes occurring in the body. The nurse does not tell the patient what to do, but fits care into the patient's context, or understanding. Patients who feel cared for feel more comfortable. They list several reasons for that feeling. Generally, feeling safe is a part of the comfort. The sense that someone understands their description of the problem and is monitoring it is a part of this feeling of safety. Providing information and demonstrating professional skills also help the patient feel safer.

Surveillance and Safety

A nurse who approaches the bedside of a sick person in an Intensive Care Unit (ICU) and briefly chats with the patient before leaving may be perceived as monitoring the person if, while chatting, the nurse's eyes rest briefly on each of the telemonitoring devices, each tube that drips, each screen that gives information. The patient realizes that the eye movements of the nurse are a part of surveillance. Nurses who are experienced and competent in their field are usually able to combine surveillance with conversation. The conversation may be related to other assessment parameters, such as symptoms experience or family changes, or the conversation may be unrelated to the patient's condition. A social experience is also a patient need. Presence forms the matrix of the whole interaction, and the feeling of safety and comfort is the outcome.

Choice

Another attribute of a relationship in which the patient can feel comfortable, cared for, and safe is the provision for autonomy. Recognizing the individual experience of the patient, giving the patient choices regarding care, and assistance with pain are all things patients have identified as essential to feeling cared for (Brown, 1986). If a relationship in which the dying patient feels cared for has been established, the patient is more willing to give control of care to others when strength and the will to make decisions diminishes. There is no need to expend energy consciously monitoring the care being given to him. The relationship is built on a trust that caregivers will respect his wishes and that the care given will be in harmony with his desires. The autonomy in this case is the ability to make a choice to continue to monitor care, or to spend energy on relationships, or to become introspective and self-focused. Trust that another person will carry out the patient's care in the preferred ways frees him to make real choices at the end of life.

Environment

Comfort for the whole person also includes care of the environment. Noxious odors, jarring noises, inappropriate lighting, crumbs in the bedclothes, absence of touch in one's life are all things that lead to discomfort. Therapeutic uses of aromas, music, touch, and other environmental components will be discussed separately.

The general principle guiding environmental care for the dying patient is to be sure that everything in the environment enhances the person's ability to use all senses. For example, lighting should be bright enough to see all hazards, such as things left on the floor or coffee tables in the path, and things that make life joyful, such as children or flowers. Music should not be so loud as to interfere with hearing other sounds, such as the doorbell or a conversation. Wrinkles in bedclothes can interfere with a person's sensations of developing skin breakdown because the wrinkles are annoying, and it is hard to differentiate them from a sore. It is important to have people in the environment. If a choice must be made between people in the environment and institutional policy or rules, the patient's goals and wishes are the guiding principles. For example, if a bone marrow transplant recipient is clearly dying, but the unit does not allow children to visit because of potential infection, the solution to the dilemma (to let the patient's children visit or not) should be made based on the patient's goals of how she wishes to die. Does she care about the potential for infection? Is she fighting for every moment of life that she can have? Or would the presence of her children be comforting, allowing her to let go of this world peacefully? Appropriate environmental control requires knowledge of the patient's goals for the end of life.

SPECIFIC AREAS OF COMFORT NEEDS

Sleep

A good night's sleep is a wonderful gift of nature. While scientists continue to try to analyze the many specific results of adequate sleep, every person can understand sleep as a restorative process. There is a reciprocal relationship between sleep and comfort. Lack of sleep leads to discomfort, and discomfort results in lack of sleep. Those treatments that lead to comfort are prerequisite for helping the patient into restorative, restful sleep.

Fear of falling asleep is a real problem for some people. Shakespeare's "to sleep, perchance to dream—aye there's the rub" is only one of many literary references to the human condition of fear of falling asleep because of nightmares or dreams. Some people fear they may not waken. Dying people sometimes lay awake for hours, imagining all sorts of terrors that might accompany the end of their lives. Their anxiety is accompanied by perspiration, tense muscles, rapid respirations, and other physiologic symptoms of anxiety that reinforce their fears of a worsening condition. Such symptoms often exacerbate the symptoms of illness, such as pain. The next day finds them unrestored, with less energy to spend in living life.

A patient who is having difficulty sleeping may have one of a number of sleep disorders. However, if the sleep problems developed only after the life-threatening illness developed, it is likely that they are related to factors such as:

- symptoms, like pain or nausea

- intense emotion, like anger or fear

- social problems, with family, job, or money

- unfamiliar environment, including a strange bed or lights

- medications or substances like alcohol or caffeine

Since dying people often experience more than one of these factors, sleep disruption is a common and very real problem for many dying patients. Avoiding as many of the factors that contribute to sleep deprivation as possible is an important part of care.

Insomnia is defined in general as a subjective complaint of poor sleep. It is subjective, because no one can determine for another whether the amount or quality of the sleep cycle is adequate. Some people normally sleep only a few hours; others sleep eight, nine, or ten hours. Rhythms of sleep vary, with some people falling asleep after midnight and waking quite refreshed seven or eight hours later. Others cannot stay awake after 9:00 P.M. Changing these patterns to fit a hospital schedule can contribute to a feeling of daytime fatigue and broken sleep. Dying people often complain of poor sleep because they have been unable to maintain their natural patterns of sleep.

Poor sleep may be divided into two parts: the inability to fall asleep, and the inability to stay asleep. An unfamiliar bed or pain at bedtime is likely to make it difficult for the patient to go to sleep. But medications or drugs, including alcohol, are more likely to cause early awakenings. Avoiding alcohol after 6:00 P.M. or rescheduling medication may be all that is required.

Some sleeplessness is concurrent with a disease, but not a part of it. For example, a menopausal woman may suffer several awakenings at night related to hot flashes. If the treatment for her illness does not prohibit the use of hormone replacement therapy, it will provide a simple solution to her problems with sleep.

Whatever the causes, lack of sleep leads to a number of outcomes that the patient would prefer to avoid. They include:

- fatigue during normal waking hours
- inability to concentrate
- irritability
- depression
- memory disturbances
- poor judgment

Physiologic changes that have been observed in people after extreme sleep deprivation also include decreased immune system function and poor wound healing (Doyle et al., 1993).

Sleep Assessment   Assessment of sleep problems begins with a clear history of past and present sleep patterns. The simple question "Do you have difficulty sleeping?" begins the assessment process, and should be asked of all people with chronic illness. If it is not asked, many people will consider sleeplessness part of the disease, and not understand that it can be treated. Further, asking "Do you have trouble falling asleep?" and "Do you wake up in the middle of the night or early in the morning?" can help in determining the cause and potential treatments.

Symptomatology that interferes with the sleep-wake cycle is assessed by asking very direct questions. Some obvious but helpful approaches are:

Do you have pain that interferes with your sleep?

Can you identify anything that keeps you from sleeping, like noise or room temperature?

Are you frightened at night?

Treatment of sleeplessness related to symptoms requires treatment of the symptoms. Similarly, if the patient can identify a medication that seems to cause sleeplessness, the need for the medication must be balanced with the need for sleep. Medications that interfere with sleep include:

- stimulants

- bronchodilators

- some antihypertensives

- activating antidepressants

- diuretics given too close to bedtime

- rebound effect from withdrawal of sedatives, hypnotics, or analgesics

- long-term opiate use, though this is not an indication to withhold pain medication

- chemicals used in society; e.g., alcohol, caffeine, and nicotine

After an initial assessment identifies the patient's perception of whether a sleep pattern disturbance exists, and the patient's identification of factors contributing to it, a more refined sleep assessment technique may be used. The use of a sleep diary documents the frequency and extent of the problem. A diary should document the sleep-wake cycle, including the sleep schedule, naps, activity, and medications used. The sleep diary should be kept for at least a week.

Sleep Hygiene Sleep hygiene is composed of two things: creation of consistent patterns of sleep behavior and creation of a sleep-conducive environment. Consistent patterns of sleep behavior means going to bed at the same time each night; maintaining as active a schedule of activity in the daytime as possible; associating bed with sleep, and staying out of it when it is not time to sleep (as a patient's condition permits); for bedridden patients, providing stimulation during the day; and avoiding naps.

Creating a sleep-conducive environment means eliminating uncomfortable things from the sleeping area, such as ticking clocks, strong odors, or air conditioners or heaters that blow directly on an individual. In the hours just before sleep, avoid caffeine and alcohol. Give diuretics in the morning rather than at night. Provide blankets if required, dim lights if appropriate, and eliminate noise. Make sure the bed sheets are clean and smooth. Some people like a special snack, like hot chocolate, warm milk, or herbal tea. While chocolate is sometimes considered to be a stimulant, if a person has been drinking it before sleep since childhood, the pattern is probably more important than the small amount of stimulant.

Sleep hygiene for the dying patient includes all of the preceding things and more. Nights are very long for people who are fearful and anxious. During the day, such anxieties are less bothersome because of distractions. At night, alone, the patient can be overwhelmed. The ability to talk with someone, psychotherapy if indicated, or the judicious use of medication may improve the ability to sleep. Medication for sleep can be counterproductive, however. As more medications are required for treatment of the illness or control of other symptoms, they may interact with drugs given to help a person sleep. When a person is weaned from the sleep medication, a rebound insomnia can occur. Medications for sleep should be given only for short periods of time, a week or two, while other therapies are tried. Pain and symptom control throughout the night are also necessary.

There are a variety of nonpharmacological treatments for insomnia that can be tried after the environment is sleep conducive and patterns of the sleep and wake cycle have been established. Behavioral treatments using standard progressive muscle relaxation, biofeedback to reduce muscle tension and stress, and brief psychotherapy to deal with fear are all helpful.

Stimulus control (the sleeper removes himself from the bed if unable to fall asleep and does something else for a while), Therapeutic Touch, and massage also seem to help.

Movement

Regular exercise is a component of good health for everyone. People vary in their individual abilities to exercise, but the benefits of regular exercise are well-known. Positive results of such simple activity as frequent posture change have been demonstrated in circulatory, respiratory, muscular, digestive, and urological systems, as well as helping to improve a person's psychological state (Doyle et al., 1993).

For the person who is dying, physical activity can help lessen pain and stiff joints, increase strength in muscles, prolong a person's ability to care for herself, and improve self-esteem. It allows the person to continue in the family role for a longer time, maintaining an optimum level of functioning. It is a component of quality of life.

Many patients who have been told that the health care system has no more to offer, that there is nothing more that can be done, feel hopeless. They give up too soon, doing less than they are able, missing many hours, days, and weeks of pleasure. Careful assessment of functional status and an understanding of the things that make life pleasant for the individual will help the nurse establish a realistic plan for mobility to help extend the pleasure in life for the patient (see "The Game Warden"). Consultation with a physical therapist may be helpful as a part of the functional assessment.

The Game Warden

Mr. Gilliard, who was from a rural area in a southern state, lived his life for hunting and fishing. As a game warden for the state, he had spent most of his life outdoors. When he was diagnosed with colon cancer and discovered that the subsequent colon resection and colostomy was not curative, he believed he would no longer hunt or fish. He became depressed, with little reason to get out of bed each day. After discharge, hospice services were arranged. The hospice nurse learned that Mr. Gilliard's satisfactions in life were outside the house, and she helped the family plan to build a path from Mr. Gilliard's home to the river bank nearby. Once he had a reason to leave his bed, get dressed, and take care of himself, he spent several peaceful and happy months providing fish and crabs for his family. It was important to the quality of his life to remain mobile, to get to the bench on the river bank to feel the breeze, hear the crickets, and watch the sunset.

Mobility Assessment Assessment of a patient for the ability to be mobile can be incorporated into a general physical assessment. Pay specific attention to areas of weakness, especially knees and ankles. Identify areas of loss of sensation, since that means the body's normal warning system is not working. If feet or hands have lost sensation because of medications that change sensorium (due to some kinds of chemotherapy, for example), they will need to be checked frequently for injury. Planned safety measures will be important, like careful reassessment of shoe size. The patient will need to avoid wearing shoes that are too tight, because the shoes may become tighter (perhaps due to edema) without the patient noticing. Skin breakdown can become quite advanced before the patient is aware of the problem, and healing can be affected, perhaps slowed due to medical treatment protocols. Include an assessment for balance and stability.

Check for dyspnea. Progressive exercise can be very helpful in improving respiratory function, but it needs to be done carefully, with clear directions to the patient. Directions must include the physician's prescription for oxygen and medication use, pursed-lip breathing, and an assessment of stamina.

A patient was asked why he sat in the house so much of the time. He answered that he was afraid if he walked down the road, he would become short of breath and would not be able to get back. Fears like this are common and may be realistic. Therefore, plans to build strength and clear directions about how

far is too far are important. Safety is a major consideration. It may
be helpful to set progressive goals—walk to the fence on day
one, to the end of the drive on day two, and so on. It may be
necessary to walk with someone the first few times. A camp stool
may be carried or a sturdy walker with wheels and a seat
attached (available commercially) may be pushed while walking,
for balance and stability. A tired person can sit on it for rest periods. Once the patient feels stronger and learns to hear what the
body is saying about fatigue, when to rest and when to go on,
a regular pattern can be established. That pattern must be
adjusted as strength fails. Pushing to meet a goal that is no longer
possible is unsafe and can lead to falls and injury. Sensitivity to
changes in physical condition is imperative, a part of competent
nursing care that involves monitoring the patient and being
present in the relationship.

Resources   There are a number of devices that help people
remain mobile longer. They include things to be carried, like
walking sticks or canes; things to be pushed, like walkers or gro-
cery carts; things to be grasped for support, like handrails or ban-
isters; and things that can carry a person, like wheelchairs.
Recliners and comfortable chairs with footstools are also helpful
aids for people if they are constructed in such a way that people can get into and out of them without undo effort. Some
patients qualify for Medicare-provided motorized recliners. They
may have seats that push the patient up and out of the chair into
a standing position. These are useful in avoiding stress in the
knees. For example, one elderly man with pronounced emphy-
sema and arthritis in both knees believes that he would be
bedridden if he did not have a chair that helps him to stand. He
can walk from the bed to a bathroom with a built-up toilet seat,
and to his special chair. This lets him care for himself and spend
time with the family in activities that they all enjoy. Without the
special recliner, he would need assistance each time he wanted
to get up.
     When continuous bedrest becomes necessary, standard
nursing techniques for position change and range of motion promote comfort. Since no one can accurately predict when a person
will die, it is not appropriate to avoid turning a person, even if
the turning is temporarily distressing, thinking that the patient will

die soon anyway. Skin breakdown can occur in a matter of hours, compounding the discomfort. The same is true of stiffening, contracting joints.

Health care is an interdisciplinary effort. Providers of care include not only medical doctors and nurses, but people like physical therapists, chiropractors, and massage therapists. Each of these disciplines can provide care that improves mobility for some people. For example, a person who has back pain or stiffness of the hips may find massage of the muscles and an exercise program planned by a physical therapist of great benefit. Simple massage, including effleurage (deep or gentle stroking) and petrissage (kneading), can easily be taught to family members as a useful aid to care (see "Mr. Bower's Back Rub"). A chiropractor may provide an adjustment that makes it possible to become more mobile than the patient had been during the acute stages of an illness. Consultation with other health care providers, when that is the patient's choice, can be useful.

Mr. Bower's Back Rub

Mr. Bower was restless, warm, and clearly uncomfortable. He did not want any pain medication. It was not that kind of pain. He was just "achy." Ms. F. said, "How about an old-fashioned back rub?" He agreed. Ten minutes later his respirations were deeper and regular, his muscles were less rigid, and he was resting in the same position for several minutes. As Ms. F. withdrew from the room, Mr. Bower's comment was, "You always seem to know what to do to make me feel more comfortable." The back rub became a standard by which to measure comfort techniques. The question "Is it as good as a back rub?" became an evaluation technique. It also became a verbal reference to a shared comfort experience that reminded them both of the caring relationship that had been established.

Touch

Touch is a basic human need. Without touch, an infant does not survive. Without touch, it is difficult to communicate love. Without touch, the elderly become withdrawn. And without touch, the dying person becomes isolated and depressed. Lack of touch is a form of sensory deprivation. Mr. Bower's back rub helped him for several reasons. The stimulation of the skin resulted in better capillary blood flow. Stimulation of nerve cells (sending rub messages rather than pain messages) blocked the perception of pain. He was also the recipient of ordinary touch.

Ordinary touch creates relationship. The skin contains millions of sensory nerve cells, and as such, is a giant organ of communication. It helps the caregiver to assess potential problems. The first indication of a fever might be simply a feeling of warm skin. Cold hands, noticed during a handshake, might indicate anxiety or that a person has just come in from the cold. The skin communicates information. Touching is a way of receiving that message.

Messages are sent through the touch of the caregiver. The nurse can send a message of security to the ill adult who is walking with an unstable gait by holding the arm firmly, not gently. Holding the arm softly while applying a lotion conveys gentleness and empathy in other circumstances.

Touching is often incidental to the act of nursing. Touch may be related to performing a procedure (e.g., giving an injection); incidental, as when a patient is too close to another person and brushes against the arm of that individual; or purposive. Purposive touch can be planned to convey a message, assess information, or facilitate social interaction. All touch seems to have some influence on people. The nurse who practices presence in patient interactions will have an awareness of the kind of message being sent and will plan the interaction of touch for appropriate outcomes. For example, a back rub in a big city hospital during evening care might seldom get done because of the real constraints of time and other duties the nurse perceives as more important. For a dying patient, a back rub could have comfort outcomes that would make the back rub a treatment rating high priority. Touch might lead to less medication, less depression, and improved sleep and mobility status. The back rub for a person who responds to it in this way should remain a part of the plan of care and receive high priority.

Appropriate outcomes of touch for the dying patient who is experiencing discomfort also include enhancement of verbal communication, facilitation of social interaction, and conveying emotion. The person who is dying is often socially isolated. Kolcaba (1992) identified four areas to address in meeting the comfort needs of dying patients. Ordinary touch meets physical, psychospiritual, and social needs, and influences environment. Touch affects every area of need.

In other eras, the dying person was hidden from view, shut off from the family or other people, and was seldom touched. A fear of touching dying people was common, and still is in some cultures. There may have been a good reason for that practice when the main cause of death was contagious disease. In fact, some HIV positive people believe that caregivers shrink back from touching them for the same reason—fear of contagion. There is no good reason for not touching the dying patient now, unless the patient chooses not to be touched for some reason.

Planned purposive touching requires careful assessment by the nurse. People learn the meaning of touch from families and culture. Hugging, for example, is expected by some as a comfort measure, but is an unwelcome intrusion to others. It is easy to ask a person, "Would you like a hug?" rather than hugging without asking. It can be uncomfortable and put up barriers to a relationship. A negative response can lead to a new question about what might help a person feel better, if not a hug. The answer might be something like, "Just sit with me for a while." The assessment prior to purposeful touch should include an honest appraisal of how comfortable the nurse is with touch, and what kinds of touch are acceptable. A sincere handshake is more likely to lead to a trusting relationship than an insincere pat on the back. For people who are clearly victims of social isolation, planning to include some sincere form of touch as often as possible is a valuable therapeutic act.

Nurses have developed or begun to use many therapeutic nursing treatments based on touch. They include:

- accupressure and Shiatzu
- Therapeutic Touch
- Reiki
- other forms of deep massage
- Traeger

Each of these treatments can be used for comfort, and each requires knowledge and practice to develop competency. They are described in detail in several places (Dossey et al., 1988; Keegan, 1994). If not taught specifically in a program of nursing, the nurse wishing to add these comfort measures to an individual practice can get a number of books from most libraries; attend certified or approved continuing education programs, or review videotapes. Be sure you can document competence in the practice of these techniques, and follow established policies within the employment setting to assure safe patient care.

SUMMARY

Planning to keep dying people comfortable is critical to helping them live with a significant quality of life near the end of life. Comfort encompasses a spectrum of feelings beginning with a sense of relief from discomfort, and ranging to a feeling of transcendence. To promote comfort, it is the nurse's responsibility to assess symptoms that cause discomfort, and the patient's ability to function at an optimum level. It is difficult for the dying patient to maintain normal comfort behaviors, like getting enough sleep, exercising, and socializing, because of the declining physical and cognitive abilities associated with the disease processes. The patient's active involvement in making choices that promote comfort, combined with the nurse's knowledge and skills in providing care, increase the patient's opportunities to achieve comfort in her last days. A simple, gentle touch helps remind a dying person that she is not alone, and she hasn't died yet!

References

Brown, L. (1986). The experience of care: patient perspectives. *Topics in Clinical Nursing, 8*(2), 56–62.

Calman, K. C. (1984). Quality of life in cancer patients—an hypothesis. *Journal of Medical Ethics, 10,* 124–127.

Dossey, B. M., Keegan, L., Guzzetta, C. E., & Kolkmeier, L. G. (1995). *Holistic nursing: A handbook for practice* (2nd ed.). Rockville, MD: Aspen Publishers, Inc.

Doyle, D., Hanks, G. W. C., & MacDonald, N. (Eds.). (1993). *Oxford textbook of palliative medicine.* Oxford: Oxford University Press.

Hines, D. R. (1987). *The concept development of presence in nursing science.* Unpublished manuscript, Texas Women's University, Denton, TX.

Hines, D. R. (1992). Presence: discovering the artistry in relating. *Journal of Holistic Nursing, 10*(4), 294–305.

Keegan, L. (1994). *The nurse as healer.* Albany, NY: Delmar Publishers.

Kolcaba, K. (1991). A taxonomic structure for the concept of comfort. *Image, 23,* 235–238.

Kolcaba, K. (1992). Holistic comfort: Operationalizing the construct as a nurse-sensitive outcome. *Advances in Nursing Science, 15,* 1–10.

McNeil, B. J., Weichselbaum, R., & Pauker, S. J. (1981). Speech and survival—trade offs between quality and quantity of life in laryngeal cancer. *New England Journal of Medicine, 305,* 982–987.

Padilla, G. V., Grant, M. M., & Ferrell, B. (1992). Nursing research into quality of life. *Quality of Life Research, 1,* 341–348.

Pettigrew, J. (1988). *A phenomenological study of the nurse's presence with persons experiencing suffering.* Unpublished doctoral dissertation, Texas Women's University, Denton, TX.

5 | PAIN MANAGEMENT

THE PROBLEM

Despite the medical and health care advances of the last two decades that have made pain controllable for most people, pain has become a reality for many. Dozens of studies have demonstrated both effective pharmacologic and nonpharmacologic pain control methods. The education of patients and caregivers alike should focus on the fact that a person does not need to live in pain. Most pain can be controlled. Initiatives to educate people about pain control come from a variety of places, including grass roots movements and the federal government. Decreasing the fear of pain helps decrease the experience (perception) of pain.

Many older people believe that pain is a fact of life with advancing years. For example, when the doctor asked one senior citizen how long his foot had been hurting, the man said five days. "Why did you wait so long before coming to see me?" asked the doctor. The old man said, "I'm old. I'm supposed to hurt!" He had been walking on a broken foot for five days.

Cultural Perceptions of Pain

A nurse asked a woman in a bush hospital if she had pain. The woman had been out of surgery for about an hour and was fully alert. Her appendectomy had been uneventful. Every 20 minutes the nurse repeated her question, expecting that the woman would soon need some pain medication. But the woman became irritated with the nurse. She said, "I only hurt where the doctor cut me!" She could not understand why the nurse would keep asking such a foolish question. Of course she had incisional pain!

Part of the terror of dying for many people is the fear of a long and wakeful night full of pain. That fear is often well-founded. Two-thirds of the patients with advanced cancer, for example, experience significant levels of pain (Ferrell et al., 1993). The fear of pain reduces the perceived quality of life, influences the ability of a person to feel comfortable, and interferes with relationships.

PAIN DEFINED

One thing on which pain experts agree is that pain is what the patient says it is. Pain is a subjective experience, involving the total person. Pain hurts. Bresler (1979) said that pain is "a sensation, an emotion, a cognition, a motivation, and an energy." How individuals perceive pain depends upon many things, including education, ethnicity, culture, physical condition, experience, severity, location, and secondary meaning.

Pain has meaning to individuals. A person who has had a serious accident involving a back injury may be relieved that pain is present, realizing that there is no spinal cord damage that would lead to permanent paralysis. Pain may be delivered by an abusive spouse, and mean fear and lack of love to the abused mate. Pain may be an expectation of changing life status, as in the old man with the broken foot. Or it may be something to warn of the need to take action. If the old man had been educated to use pain as a warning to take action, he probably would have seen the doctor earlier. Pain can be useful.

Dying people often see pain as deterioration in physical condition. This may or may not be real. Abdominal pain in a dying patient may be related to the illness, or it may be a new problem that can be treated. Constipation, for example, is a common problem for people on multiple medications, with little activity and poor appetite. Constipation can cause abdominal pain. If the health care provider believes that the complaint of abdominal pain for this person is a new stage in the disease progression, steps to relieve the constipation may be delayed and suffering experienced. All complaints of pain should be assessed adequately.

Mr. Bower's Pain

Mr. Bower sat smoking in the solarium, unable to sleep, unable to pace the way he usually did while waiting for Ms. F. to talk with him. She asked him if he was in pain, and he said no. However, he grimaced and winced every time he adjusted his position.

Finally, she asked him why he did not take the medicine prescribed for his pain. Mr. Bower answered that the longer he postponed the medicine, the better it would work when he really needed it. Ms. F. explained that it did not work that way. She taught him to ask for the medicine before the pain got bad, and told him of newer pain control measures that would be available when he needed them. Three nights later, he thanked her. He was much more comfortable.

ASSESSMENT

Adequate and continuing assessment of pain requires three things. The first is recognition of the fact that a person perceives pain to be present. The second is documentation of pain treatment. Documentation of the progress/relief of the pain is the third. Many studies have shown that barriers to effective pain management include the fact that professional caregivers, including physicians and nurses, consistently underestimate pain and either underprescribe or inadequately medicate patients who need pain medication. Patients do not report pain in a timely way, preferring to wait until it is severe for many reasons. The reasons may include culturally learned responses to pain; fear of becoming addicted; and not understanding when optimum pain control measures should be started. In addition, there is little attention given to nonpharmacologic treatments that have been shown to be effective in the relief of mild to moderate pain, or that potentiate the action of medication for all levels of pain. The first step in changing the inadequacy of pain management is to assess it realistically.

Professional caregivers are likely to rely on their own assessment of health status for most patient problems. Clinical decision making is taught in professional schools with an emphasis on objective evidence, with subjective reports often considered unimportant. The only reliable report of the existence of pain is subjective. Pain cannot be seen or objectively measured. The assessment of pain must be done first by the patient, and even unreliable historians or confused people should be believed about the presence and extent of their pain.

There are many good assessment tools that can be adapted to individual situations. Assessment tools are helpful in reminding caregivers what to assess regarding pain, and to keep an ongoing record of pain history, management, and outcome of treatment.

Interview

The first kind of assessment that should be done is a structured interview in which the person with pain is asked to tell about her pain. After determining that the person perceives pain to be present, ask how it was managed previously, what kind of pain treatments help or do not help, and what kind of advice the person would give to a friend or family member in a similar situation (Ferrell et al., 1993). This kind of information gives the caregiver insight into how aggressively the patient is able to manage self-care. The acceptability and usefulness of different types of treatments are also identified in the interview. The patient can decide when to start a new course of treatment because the old one is not working. When the patient feels someone is listening to an important problem, it helps the relationship between nurse and patient and gives hope that the problem can be managed. Since most pain can be managed, that hope should be supported and encouraged.

The information from the structured interview can be recorded with more specific data on an initial pain assessment tool. This data includes location, intensity, degree of distress, quality of the pain (sharp pain or aches, for example), when it started, and how long it usually lasts (McCaffrey & Beebe, 1989). Location of pain can easily be detected by asking the patient to mark a drawing of a person in the places where pain exists.

Rating Scales

Pain rating scales for pain intensity and pain distress are illustrated in figure 5.1. In lieu of the pain rating scales presented, a person can be asked to rate pain using a number from 0–10, with zero indicating no pain, and 10 the worst possible pain. Whether a written pain rating scale or the choice of a number to indicate intensity of pain is used, it should be consistently used with each patient, and written on a flow sheet so that the pattern of pain intensity can be traced over time. This allows the nurse to evaluate pain management strategies. The form is used to record regular assessments of pain intensity, treatments used for pain control, and has columns for other relevant information (Faries et al., 1991). Figure 5.2 illustrates how a flow sheet to record pain intensity and treatment might be set up for Mrs. Foote.

Mrs. Foote is a 43-year-old patient with cervical cancer who was admitted to the hospital to develop pain management

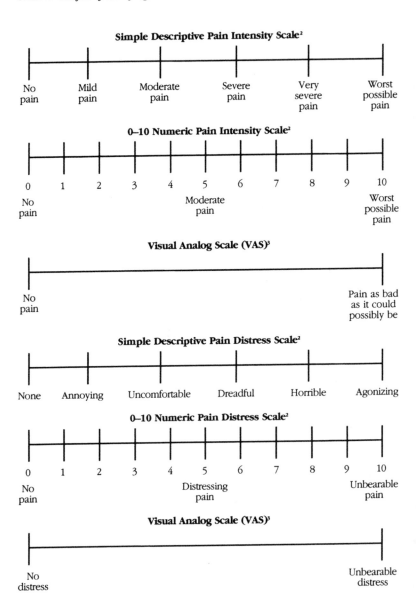

FIGURE 5.1 Comparison of Pain Intensity and Pain Scales[1]

[1]Acute Pain Management Guideline Panel. *Acute Pain Management: Operative or Medical Procedures and Trauma. Clinical Practice Guideline.* AHCPR Pub. No. 92-0032. Rockville, MD: Agency for Health Care Policy and Research, Public Health Service, U.S. Department of Health and Human Services. February 1992.

[2]If used as a graphic rating scale, a 10 cm baseline is recommended.

[3]A 10 cm baseline is recommended for VAS scales.

ASSESSMENT				MEDICINE	PCA		OTHER	
Date/ Time	Sed. Level	Resp. Rate	*Pain Rating	Analgesic: Drug/Dose/Route	Bolus; Shift	Shift Drug Total	**Nonpharm Therapies	Plan/ Signature

Sedation Level:
  0—Fully alert
  1—Relaxed, awake
  2—Drowsy, dozing
  3—Arousable sleep
  4—Unarousable

FIGURE 5.2   *Flow Sheet, Pain Control*

*Pain Rating: Use Scale of 0–10, 0 = no pain; 10 = severe pain.
**Nonpharm Therapies = heat, cold, relaxation techniques, imagery, and so on.
Adapted from Faries et al., 1991.

strategies. She is in the late stages of her disease and is planning to return home to die if the pain can be controlled there. During the hospital visit, she will be taught the use of a patient-controlled analgesia device (PCA) using opiates, guided imagery to potentiate the action of the medications, and when to ask for changes in protocol. Professional staff will titrate the appropriate dosages of both the opiates and the nonsteroidal antiinflammatory drugs (NSAIDs) based on her assessment of pain intensity. All of these things could be done at home, but her physician is also evaluating the need for further radiation treatments, and if the pain control is inadequate, anesthesia techniques for pain control. Because Mrs. Foote has determined that one of her important goals is to remain alert, the flow sheet has a column to assess her level of alertness during the evaluation process. Because respiratory distress and constipation are potential side-effects of the opiates used, the flow sheet also has space to evaluate them.

The flow sheet used for her should be continued at home by home health, hospice, or family caregivers. She may be stable for a long period of time, but occasionally suffer from *breakthrough pain.* That is the term given to a transitory exacerbation of pain even though adequately controlled most of the time. Such pain is usually managed with additional medication, which may be needed for only a short period of time. Should a pattern of breakthrough pain be identified, she may want to learn cognitive strategies for dealing with the fear of such pain recurring. This is the time to use relaxation techniques (so that tense muscles do not increase painful stimuli) or imagery in which she could recall the feelings of security provided by a safe or peaceful place. Fear and peace do not coexist. Pain management protocols should be reevaluated if the breakthrough pain becomes a pattern.

The choice of a consistent method of rating pain intensity should be a policy decision of the institution or agency caring for patients in pain. That allows for adequate education of the staff concerning the meaning of pain intensity scales, resulting in more consistent pain management for the patients.

A Child's Pain

Children need a different way of assessing pain. Studies to learn the best way of measuring a child's pain are underway by a variety of researchers. Some use a poker chip strategy in which a child is given four red poker chips and taught to describe pain in terms of the number of chips, or "pieces of pain," experienced right now (Acute Pain Management Guideline Panel, 1992). Others use a series of simple faces, the first face smiling, the last one crying, and two or three in the middle in various states of unhappiness. The child is asked to point to the face that shows how the pain makes him feel right now. The child can be told if there is no hurt to point to the smiling face, if there is enough hurt to be a little unhappy to point to the next face, and so on. Once pain has been identified as present using this technique, the nurse can get even a small child to begin to talk about the hurt with such statements as, "Oh! You have a little hurt. Tell me about your little hurt. Point to your little hurt." The child can also be asked what the nurse should do to relieve the pain. Sometimes a hug is all that is required, but a big hurt will not be so easily treated. It is important to recognize that children do have pain, and it should be treated appropriately. Living with pain slows the healing process, causes distrust of the nurse and doctor, and diminishes quality of life for children, even as it does for adults.

THEORIES OF PAIN

By far the most common theory used to guide treatment of the patient in pain is the gate control theory. Knowledge of the physiological transmission of pain is the foundation on which the theory is built.

Transmission of Pain

Pain is transmitted from nocioceptors, cells that respond to injury or painful stimuli. When nocioceptors are injured, they release chemical substances that initiate the pain impulses and mediate pain responses. Nocioceptors are located on the ends of neurons, nerve cells. Three types of neurons involved in transmission of pain are sensory neurons, efferent or motor neurons, and connector neurons.

Peripheral nerve fibers are of different sizes, and conduct sensation differently. Sensory (afferent) impulses are conducted by the peripheral nerve fibers to the dorsal horn of the spinal cord. Chemicals, including neurotransmitters like acetylcholine, dopamine, epinephrine, and norepinephrine, help the impulse over the synapse (the space between ends of nerves). The impulse is conducted to the opposite side of the spinal cord, and travels along the spinothalamic tract to the higher centers in the brain. Some centers in the brain that are directly involved in perception of pain include the thalamus, hypothalamus, brain stem, and cortex. Within each of these areas there is a variety of functions, including memory, interpretation of signals, and emotional response. They are all involved in the transmission of pain (McGuire, 1994).

The gate-control theory of pain proposes that a mechanism to inhibit painful sensory impulses exists within the spinal cord, in an area called the substantia gelatinosa. That mechanism is called a gate, and it can be closed to pain impulses by stimulating nerve fibers that carry other sensations, like touch or temperature. This is not an all or none phenomenon. In general, if many fibers of one kind are stimulated, fewer impulses get through using the other fibers. But the touch and temperature transmissions do not last long, and pain can quickly become the dominant impulse. In addition, the noxious stimuli can stimulate many more fibers that carry pain, and overwhelm the system so that touch and temperature do not get through. The theory explains why we can rub a sore area to make it feel better. We stimulate the touch sensory fibers and that decreases the pain for a short time. The usefulness of ice to numb a painful area is also partially explained by the gate control theory. The gate control theory is useful in suggesting several methods of pain control. Local anesthesia that stops the initial transmission of pain, or treatments that set up competition between fibers that carry pain and fibers that carry other messages in the nervous system (like ice and cold on a painful area or massage of a sore muscle) are explained in part by this theory.

Other ways of inhibiting pain use chemicals found in the nervous system. Endorphins are large polypeptides found in the pituitary and other places within the central nervous system (CNS) which prevent conduction of pain impulses within the CNS. They are naturally occurring substances with morphine-like qualities. Enkephalins are smaller neurotransmitters that close the pain gate by binding with opiate receptors in the dorsal horn of the spinal cord, thus preventing the transmission of the pain impulse. Chemicals (medications) of various types can be used to stop or change the perception of pain, both in the peripheral nervous system and in the CNS.

Perception of Pain

Because centers of memory, emotion, and learning are involved in the transmission of pain, they influence the perception of pain. For example, if a patient remembers that a particular kind of pain went away quickly in the past, there will be less emotion, less muscle tensing, and less fear than if the type of pain currently experienced reminds her of a prolonged, serious, and debilitating illness. If a person can focus, perhaps through guided imagery or another cognitive technique, on feeling safe and comfortable, pain may not intrude.

When pain becomes a severe problem for a dying patient, the use of a combination of treatments is advocated. There are many ways to close the gate to the transmission of pain. One way is seldom sufficient because there are so many fibers and so many components of the pain system that a single treatment aimed at one part of the system can be overwhelmed. A variety of treatments support each other.

PHARMACOLOGIC TREATMENT OF PAIN

Standards of pain control treatment suggest that moderate to severe pain usually requires some type of medication for adequate control. The huge variety of medication available, the multiplicity of administration techniques, and the potentially serious nature of side effects make decisions about the best method of pain control for an individual patient a difficult task for the health care provider. While the primary physician or nurse practitioner generally is responsible for the order for medication, the patient, nurse, and family provide information upon which to base the decision, and are often given the choice between doses and types of medications to be used within guidelines. It is very important that everyone who has a role in the management of a patient's pain be clear about the patient's goals and the principles of pharmacologic pain management.

Appendix 1 reprints the dosage charts for different types of pharmacologic pain control for acute pain in adults and children (Acute Pain Management Guideline Panel, 1992). These dosage charts are a helpful place to start, recognizing that a combination of these drugs will provide a combination of sites of action and increase the potential for pain relief. For example, it is possible to pick a nonsteroidal antiinflammatory medication with a site of action in the peripheral nervous system and an opiate that works centrally, thereby combining the effects of the drugs to prevent transmission of pain impulses in both areas. Dosages presented in the table are a place to start titrating medication needed for pain control, recognizing that much larger doses may be required for patients in severe, chronic pain. Patients who are dying may need treatment for acute pain when undergoing diagnostic procedures, recovering from surgery, or recovering from trauma or complications of disease, like fractures sustained during a fall. It is not reasonable to assume that because treatment is given for chronic pain, the same treatment will relieve acute pain. New pains need to be reassessed, and goals reevaluated.

Additives and Adjuvants

Some medications are commonly used to combat side effects of the pain or other medication. These medications may be added to the pain control protocols, and are sometimes called additives. They are different from adjuvant medications which potentiate the action of the main analgesic. Examples of adjuvant drugs include caffeine or tricyclic antidepressants, which are used to stimulate or change the depressive action of some opioids, making the opioid more effective. Phenergan is an example of a drug used by many nurses to potentiate the action of Demerol, although it is now thought to have no analgesia potentiating effects (McGuire, 1994). It can still be combined with Demerol to treat nausea and vomiting, and so is an additive.

Complications

Chronic pain is different from acute pain. The length of time the pain lasts, the progression of the disease process, and the development of some tolerance for medication require constant reassessment of the efficacy of the treatment being given. There are some principles to keep in mind when reassessing pain management strategies.

Less than one percent of people who take opiates for the relief of chronic pain become addicted to the medication (Ferrell et al., 1991). Addiction seldom occurs in this population when pain is present. For many nurses, the fear that patients will become addicted to pain medication is a factor in choosing whether to give the medication. *Pain medication should not be withheld or given sparingly for people who have chronic pain because of an unfounded fear of addiction.* Patients who are addicted to narcotics or other pain medications before the problems with pain related to an illness begin may pose some difficult treatment decisions because the doses of medications required to adequately treat the pain will seem high. It is necessary to work with the person in pain to achieve the best possible pain relief. Everyone has the right to adequate pain control if it is possible.

One well-known complication of narcotics is the potential for respiratory depression. Some nurses are afraid to give the high dose of narcotics required to control pain because they believe that high doses of narcotics will compromise the patient's respiratory status. Research has shown, however, that respiratory depression is seldom a complication of narcotics administration if the patient has been requiring increasing amounts of the medication to control pain. It seems that the same mechanisms that lead to tolerance of the effects of the medication with regard to pain control also lead to tolerance with regard to respiratory depression. Of course, respiratory status must be monitored as it would be for all patients taking narcotics.

For the few people who do experience respiratory depression resulting from the only medication that relieves pain for them, giving the medication may pose an ethical dilemma. That dilemma is resolved by clarity of patient goals and organizational policy. If the patient's goal is to be comfortable, and the organization's policies permit it, the medication may be given. The patient and/or family should understand the consequences of giving the medication, including side effects. It should be clear that the medication is given for pain control, not to shorten life, though that may occur. If the patient's goal is for the longest life span possible, that person may choose to endure the pain rather than take the risk of dying. The nurse will continue to seek all available pain control treatments. A nurse who has a moral or ethical belief that makes it impossible to administer a medication for relieving pain when that medication may result in complications like respiratory depression will need to make other arrangements to help the patient achieve goals for a peaceful, pain-free death. A supervisor can help. Narcotics are not administered to shorten a life. That is euthanasia, which is illegal in the United States.

Timing of Administration

Prevention of severe pain is more useful than treating it after it becomes severe. Consequently, it is important for members of the pain treatment team to understand that medication must be given before the pain becomes severe. Waiting until the pain recurs as an indicator of need for analgesia may be too late. Current pain control standards recommend the use of regular, around-the-clock administration of the medication. Monitoring the patient for appropriate dosage includes the level of pain, vital signs, level of consciousness, related symptoms like nausea or confusion, and reporting the response of nonpharmacological pain control strategies.

A patient who has chronic, severe pain generally needs a medication that is released into the body continuously, rather than intermittently. This keeps the level of medication and the pain in balance, and the person can maintain a low pain (or pain-free) lifestyle. Recent technological developments have made this possible. Sustained-release oral medications and the transdermal patch are two examples. One goal of ongoing research in this field is to be able to offer a variety of medications that are continuously released to relieve pain more consistently.

Methods of Administration

Oral   As a rule of thumb, oral administration of medications is preferred as the least invasive, easiest, and most cost-effective means of delivering medication. Some oral medications are available as controlled-release preparations. Morphine, for example, can be given orally in a controlled-release formula that reaches its peak action in two to four hours, but maintains a constant plasma level for about twelve hours. A twice-a-day regimen can keep patients who respond to oral morphine comfortable more easily than repeated injections or four hourly tablets. However, there are many reasons why moderate-to-severe chronic pain may not respond well to oral administration of pain medication. Some medications are not well-absorbed in the gastrointestinal tract. Some cause side effects like nausea and vomiting. Sometimes a sick patient has problems swallowing or digesting anything, including medications. When oral administration is not possible, there are many other routes of administration of pain medication.

Rectal or Sublingual For medications that are absorbable in the G.I. tract, rectal or sublingual administration may be an option. These are usually temporary measures, and are dependent upon the patient not having diarrhea, sores in the mouth, or other digestive tract disturbances that cause discomfort. If it is likely that the pain is not going away, but will become chronic, and the oral route is no longer available, a more dependable route that assures the same amount of absorption of the medication during each administration will be used.

Transdermal Patch One area of significant development is the transdermal patch. Fentanyl can be administered in this way. Transdermal patches are adhesive patches with medication in the center. They release medication through the skin continuously, as long as the patch is in place. This maintains a constant level of the medication to keep a person comfortable. Care of a person using a patch includes the assessment of the level of pain control, the maintenance of a pain flow sheet, and the administration of a rapidly absorbed pain medicine for breakthrough pain, should that occur. Skin care is important, and should be given according to directions that come with the patches. The old medication is usually removed, and the new patch placed in a different area.

Intravenous Continuous Opioid Infusion (ICOI) Another method of continuous administration of medication (specifically opioids like morphine) is an infusion pump. The pump is set to deliver the medication continuously. An alarm should be used to warn of changes in rate of infusion or an empty chamber. When a patient is first started on ICOI, it is important to monitor vital signs and other parameters of safety every 15 minutes for two hours and until they are stable. Record the results on a flow sheet.

Patient-Controlled Analgesia (PCA)   When the PCA pump is used, medication is released intravenously each time the patient pushes the button on the syringe pump mechanism. The medication may be in a cartridge-like reservoir located on a pump through which a regular I.V. is set up. Another option is a small, portable unit that can be attached to the wrist and easily carried around. The pump always has a series of safety devices to prevent accidental administration of medication, including a lockout mechanism which prevents a second dose from being given within five to twenty minutes of the previous dose. The PCA pump gives the patient the control in treating pain. The patient is encouraged to self-medicate via a patient-controlled analgesia pump before the pain becomes severe. Waiting does not diminish the need, and additional medication may be required if the pain gets out of control.

A nurse who is caring for a patient using any mechanical devices must be completely familiar with them, including how to set them up, safety mechanisms, potential dangers, and side effects of the medication. Standard care of the I.V. site is required, with special care for patients with poor venous access, to preserve the veins adequate for infusion purposes. Caring for patients who are on narcotics at home requires a thorough understanding of the narcotic laws of the state, and requirements for documentation of drug use and waste disposal of them.

Spinal Anesthesia and Nerve Blocks   Epidural anesthesia is the infusion of an anesthetic agent, such as morphine, into the epidural space via a small catheter. Spinal anesthesia can also be given by using the subarachnoid space (intrathecal administration of medication). In both cases, the medication can be given by bolus or by continuous infusion pump. An anesthesiologist inserts the catheter and administers the first dose of medication. In addition to monitoring the patient's pain and titrating the amounts of medication needed, the nurse has several other responsibilities when caring for a patient being medicated in these ways.

Complications of this method of pain control include the potential eroding of the epidural catheter into the subarachnoid space. This is likely to result in respiratory depression because of the larger dose of medication used in the epidural route infusing into the subarachnoid space, in effect causing an overdose. Infection at the insertion site and erosion of catheters into blood vessels are also potential complications. Special in-service instruction related to techniques of administration and potential complications of these forms of medication administration is required. Some policies call for apnea monitors, as well as frequent visual monitoring.

Nerve blocks interrupt the transmission of nervous impulses by injection of local anesthetic or neurolytic agent into or around a peripheral or sympathetic/parasympathetic nerve route. Local anesthetics are short term and easily reversible medications. Neurolytic agents are permanent, used as a chemical interruption in pain pathways. They are only done after careful explanation, trials with other forms of pain control, and for severe pain.

Most people recognize a local nerve block from a visit to the dentist. Dentists frequently use nerve blocks prior to potentially painful procedures. Nerve blocks for pain control can be done by local infiltration, or injection into nerves or ganglia. A sympathetic nerve block is done by injection of local anesthetic or neurolytic agent into the spinal cord. Nerve blocks can cause allergic reactions, numbness and loss of both sensory and motor function, weakness of the part of the body affected, even hypotension. This form of pain control is usually used for a short time. If it is effective, a permanent interruption in the pain pathway may be made by surgical incision to provide long-term pain relief.

NONPHARMACOLOGIC TREATMENT OF PAIN

Surgical intervention, electrical stimulation, physical stimulation, acupuncture, Therapeutic Touch, and behavioral/cognitive techniques are all useful in the treatment of pain. They may be combined with pharmacologic methods of pain control, or in some cases used alone.

Surgical Intervention

Surgical intervention for pain control involves the interruption of nerve pathways in either the peripheral nerves, spinal cord, or brain. These techniques are used for people who are not expected to die very soon, because the disruption in their lives caused by the surgery limits the usefulness. For the person with intractable pain, whose disease is expected to be in remission for a time, or for whom no other treatment has worked, surgery may be considered.

Acupuncture

Like surgery, acupuncture may be considered an invasive pain control method because it involves the use of thin needles inserted into specific acupuncture points in the body. These points occur along meridians, channels through which energy flows in the body, according to Chinese theory. The mechanism by which this occurs is not well-defined.

Although all practitioners do not agree about the mechanism of action of acupuncture (how it works), there is agreement that it does work for many people. It replaces chemical anesthesia for many people in China, and is used in pain control clinics around the world for chronic pain like that of arthritis and herpes zoster (shingles). Acupuncture has few side effects, and is economical and efficient. It may not be as popular in the U.S. as in Asia because of easier access to chemical products and drugs. Standardized dosages for drugs makes outcomes somewhat predictable. Acupuncture and other pain control measures that are noninvasive but related (like Shiatsu) are often dependent upon the skill of the practitioner and individual differences among patients. Practitioners of acupuncture are now regulated in about half of the states.

Noninvasive Pain Control

Margo McCaffrey, a nurse, is a major advocate and researcher in the field of pain control. She has developed several guidelines to use whenever noninvasive pain control techniques are a part of the nursing care plan. They include:

- Obtain a doctor's order for techniques not clearly within the scope of independent nursing practice.

- Educate all caregivers (health care team and family) about the purpose, frequency, and specific skills needed to implement the technique.
- Individualize the technique for the patient.
- Teach and have the patient practice techniques before they are needed.
- Start the technique for pain control before the pain begins or as soon as possible after it starts.

McCaffrey also emphasizes the use of the nurse-patient relationship in assessing the patient's acceptance of the planned techniques, willingness to learn and practice, and the general acceptability of the method (McCaffrey, 1979). Mrs. Foote, who was introduced earlier, was taught to use guided imagery for pain control because that was her choice. Other options might have included progressive relaxation or hypnosis.

Electrical Stimulation

Electrical stimulation is usually delivered by a portable device called a transcutaneous electrical nerve stimulator (TENS). It uses two to four electrode patches attached to a small, battery-operated box that delivers a mild electrical stimulation to the skin near the painful area. The patient can control the intensity, rate, and duration of the stimulation. The electrical stimulation is thought to work by stimulating the large nerve fibers, closing the gate of pain transmission. There are some preliminary data that suggest electrical stimulation might speed healing, especially of bone fractures. The mechanism for this is not clear and the studies are ongoing.

The patient who will use TENS for pain management needs to learn several skills, including skin care and care of the unit and batteries. TENS will be incorporated into the total plan of care. The electrodes should be applied near the site of the pain, but avoiding any broken or reddened areas of skin, eyes, or the carotid sinuses. The use of hypoallergenic tape to avoid skin breakdown is suggested. While applying or removing the electrodes, the unit is in the off position. Once the electrodes are taped in place, the controls are increased in intensity until a mild, pleasant, local sensation is experienced. That sensation is sometimes described as tingling or buzzing, or even as gentle rain

(McGuire, 1994). If it is uncomfortable or if muscle contractions are evident, the unit should be turned down.

Units vary, and the user should follow the manufacturer's instructions for care of the unit and controls. Batteries must be recharged on a regular schedule. Patients with other battery-operated devices, such as cardiac pacemakers and implantable cardiac defibrillators, are not candidates for TENS.

Obviously, the patient using TENS must be able to follow directions. As with other noninvasive pain management strategies, the TENS unit should be used before pain becomes severe.

Physical Stimulation

Physical stimulation techniques for pain control include application of heat and cold, and various forms of massage. Both heat and cold decrease pain by stimulating pain transmission fibers, and they both decrease muscle spasms. Heat tends to bring blood flow to an area, thereby increasing edema. Cold decreases blood flow to an area, decreasing edema and hemorrhage. Cold is also useful in decreasing itching, a common problem with people who are receiving many medications or who are in bed for long periods of time.

Mr. Bower's back rub (see chapter 4) is the simplest example of effective massage. Using gentle stroking and kneading movements, the nurse stimulates peripheral nerves, limiting the use of those nerves for carrying pain messages. At the same time, the meaning of the act for Mr. Bower was that caring occurred, and that thought distracted him from the constancy of his discomfort.

Hand massage and foot massage are useful in accomplishing the same goals. The act of touching establishes connection with the patient. Foot and hand massage distract from the pain, and increase comfort. Some nurses practice reflexology, a technique of foot massage in which specific points on the foot are thought to correlate with different parts of the body. No physical connection has yet been established, but some patients report that reflexology makes them more relaxed and relieves their pain.

Shiatsu, a form of acupressure, is another specialized form of massage that may be useful in pain management. The practitioner uses the fingers, thumbs, and heels of the hand to press on the acupuncture points, rather than inserting needles (Dossey et al., 1988). It is used in Japan primarily to maintain health rather than treat illness. It is a general pain management strategy rather than a specific technique for a specific pain. This technique requires special training.

Therapeutic Touch (TT)

This technique also requires some special training, and is useful for relaxation, decreasing anxiety, and pain management. Developed by a nurse (Delores Krieger, RN, PhD, of New York University), it has rapidly gained popularity in the last 15 years. Because it is based on the theory that people are fields of energy, Therapeutic Touch (TT) can be used as a nontouch technique without losing its effectiveness. This works because the toucher is working in the energy field that extends beyond the body. In the vignette about Judy, the use of the nontouch method of TT is described.

Judy

Judy was a 25-year-old woman who was admitted to the burn unit of a large hospital with burns over 95 percent of her body. She died six weeks later. During that time, she was subjected to the standard treatments for severe burns, including large amounts of fluid, hydrotherapy, dressing changes that were excruciatingly painful, and multiple medications. It was always considered likely that she would die. The constant pain required large amounts of pain medication. The medication was partially effective but left Judy with the inability to concentrate, confusion, and insomnia. She was very frightened. Asked if she would like to try Therapeutic Touch to help her be less anxious and possibly help with the pain, she agreed. The nurse followed the five steps of TT:

- centered herself
- assessed the energy field, looking for areas of imbalance or blockage of energy flow

- "unruffled" the field
- modulated the energy
- grounded Judy

The TT treatments were done just before dressing changes, or before Judy wanted to go to sleep. She began to relax a little, and learned to practice breathing techniques to assist in relaxation so that she could control her ability to relax. While the dressing changes continued to be painful, she was able to cooperate so they could be done efficiently. She was able to say good-bye to her loved ones and write her will. She died of infection.

There is an increasing body of research that documents the effectiveness of TT. Nurses are using it whenever anxiety interferes with a patient's ability to understand and make choices, as well as a part of pain management. When it is not a part of the basic nursing curriculum, it is taught as a continuing education offering or in workshops around the country. The practice of TT is dependent upon one's ability to center. The practice of centering (a meditative awareness of self and the environment) helps and sometimes changes the nurse as much as it does the patient. Nurses report feeling calmer and less stressed after practicing TT, more satisfied with their ability to care for people. It is an example of two people (patient and nurse) in one energy field changed by conscious intention for the good of both people. As such, it is similar to the practice of healers from a variety of cultures, in which relationship is the core of healing. It is often taught to family members who wish to share this experience with a loved one.

Behavioral/Cognitive Interventions

These interventions are useful for the patient who is willing and able to learn self-regulation techniques to help control pain. Visualization, imagery, and relaxation are effective tools for the patient to learn. They are useful in the control of mild to moderate pain, and to potentiate pain medications when pain is severe.

Progressive muscle relaxation (PMR) is the most widely recognized and used technique of this kind. The patient alternately tenses and relaxes parts of the body in order, either from toe to head or head to toe, focusing on the difference in the feeling of tenseness and relaxation. After some practice, the tensing part of the exercise can be omitted because the patient knows what relaxed muscles feel like. Fifteen to 20 minutes practice three times a day prepares the patient to use this technique before and after painful events (following procedures, after treatments like radiation or surgery, and so on). Teaching patients relaxation before they need to use it for pain control is important.

When teaching relaxation, a quiet environment and comfortable position in which the spine is supported in good alignment are helpful. Background noise should be kept to a minimum, or soft music of a kind that the patient enjoys may be used to distract attention from the noise. It is not necessary to cultivate a special type of speaking voice. A regular, medium-paced delivery of a scripted message is helpful. Three scripts for different types of relaxation are printed in the government guidelines for treatment of acute pain (Acute Pain Management Guideline Panel, 1992). Once the patient has learned the script, music can be delivered through headphones to block out noise. A relaxation script can also be delivered by audiocassette tape. This is a useful way of encouraging home practice.

Once a person has learned some form of relaxation, visualization or guided imagery is a logical next step. The nurse can be creative in developing pain management strategies using visualization as long as a few basic rules are followed. They include planning the script ahead of time, using images with which the patient is familiar, following the principles of physiology when creating images, and beginning sessions with relaxation. For specific pain management, images might include a peaceful scene. Peace is a feeling that is usually incompatible with pain. For example, one person with an injured, painful hand imagined himself on the bank of a stream with his hand dangling in the water. Words that included all the senses, like a cool feeling in the hand, green color and pine smell of the woods, babbling sounds and fresh taste of the spray of water from the stream, created a sensation of peace that distracted him from the pain. The feeling of coolness on the hand in the image may also have altered the perception of pain in the brain, helping to limit the noxious sensations. At the end of the visualization session, he told himself his hand would remain cool and almost numb. For two hours after the session, he remained almost pain-free, and was able to enjoy visiting with his family.

For people who have not been taught the use of visualization or relaxation preparatory to painful procedures or the onset of pain related to disease, it is still possible to achieve relaxation. Starting with simple breathing techniques, even a yawn, and using times while the pain is not severe for practice, the patient can learn to relax and imagine. If using PMR, it is probably wise to avoid the tensing phase if the patient is in pain. One way of initiating the process and achieving almost instant results for some people is to combine methods. Using TT to help the patient become relaxed, then leading an imagery exercise is a useful combination.

CREATIVE ARTS

The use of other forms of cognitive and behavioral therapies to help manage pain is limited only by one's creativity. Hospitals now have humor carts, which are described in chapter 6. There are contests for funniest contributions to the carts. A good laugh provides a deep breath, distraction from the pain of the moment, and perhaps some endorphin release. The patient does not feel pain as deeply when laughing.

A loved pet, perhaps a cat curled up and purring next to a person in pain, is an essential part of that person's healing relationships. An old, loved hound who presents his head to be stroked helps a person recall times of joy, lessening the pain of the moment. For a person who is dying, the comfort, the touch of an animal may be as important as the touch of another person. The knowledge that the animal will be cared for after the owner's death is also vital to a sense of well-being.

Art is a useful tool in pain management. A child of six was asked to draw her pain. When it took the form of a fire, and the drawing included firefighters putting water on the blaze, the nurse suggested that ice might help the child's pain. The ice pack provided immediate relief for a time, and the child was delighted that the nurse had used "her idea." Adults sometimes use drawing in a symbolic way. It became routine for one man to draw his pain in an elaborate context, very dark, very structured, very detailed. He then cut it to shreds with scissors.

Humor, pets, art, and music therapy are all examples of creative avenues to explore for people dealing with pain. Most can be used within the context of a healing relationship, demonstrating a sense of care for the dying individual. Sometimes they can be used to assess pain, suggest management strategies, distract and change pain perception, and relieve anger. The relief of anger is important, in part because angry people so often tense muscles and move into rigid postures. Relieving the anger may relieve some tensing, which in turn relieves pain.

SUMMARY

Pain is a subjective experience. Many dying people will experience some degree of pain related to their disease process. They should know that it is not necessary to continue to live with pain. Most pain can be managed.

Pain has meaning to people. This chapter did not address the kind of pain that comes with loss, depression, or lack of meaning in life. But the physical pain that comes with disease contributes to those other kinds of pain, intensifying it and causing suffering. The combination of effective pain control and healing relationships helps to decrease that suffering.

References

Acute Pain Management Guideline Panel. (1992). *Acute pain management: Operative or medical procedures and trauma. Clinical practice guideline.* (AHCPR Publication No. 92-0032). Rockville, MD: Agency for Health Care Policy and Research, Public Health Service, U.S. Department of Health and Human Services.

Bresler, D. (1979). *Free yourself from pain.* New York: Simon and Schuster, Inc.

Dossey, B., Keegan, L., Guzzetta, C., & Kolkmeier, L. (1995). *Holistic nursing: A handbook for practice* (2nd ed.) Rockville, MD: Aspen Publishers, Inc.

Faries, J. E., Mills, D. S., Goldsmith, K. W., Phillips, K. D., & Orr, J. (1991). Systematic pain records and their impact on pain control. *Cancer Nursing, 14*(6), 306–313.

Ferrell, B., Eberts, M., McCaffery, M., & Grant, M. (1991). Clinical decision making and pain. *Cancer Nursing, 14*(6), 289–297.

Ferrell, B., Taylor, E., Grant, M., Fowler, M., & Corbisiero, R. (1993). Pain management at home: struggle, comfort, and mission. *Cancer Nursing, 16*(3), 169–178.

McCaffrey, M. (1979). *Nursing management of the patient with pain* (2nd ed.). Philadelphia: JB Lippincott, Co.

McCaffrey, M., & Beebe, A. (1989). *Pain: Clinical manual for nursing practice.* St. Louis: C.V. Mosby.

McGuire, L. (1994). Pain. In P. Beare & J. Meyers (Eds.), *Principles and practices of adult health nursing* (pp. 247–276) (2nd ed.). St. Louis: C.V. Mosby.

6

CARE OF THE PERSON WHO IS FRIGHTENED

THE PROBLEM

Anxiety accompanies many of life's changes. Approaching death is one of those changes. A common way of looking at anxiety is to consider it a general state of discomfort stimulated by new experiences. Fear is a kind of anxiety that is more focused, less general than anxiety. For example, a person is anxious about something going wrong, but fearful about an infiltrating I.V. Mrs. Nolan experienced a debilitating anxiety.

Mrs. Nolan

In the late 1960s, Mrs. Nolan visited her sick friend Mary every day until she died. The death was a hard one. Mary was in pain that was not well-controlled. Her room smelled bad, a foul smell that many believed to be characteristic of cancer. Mary cried a lot and could do nothing for herself, not even let go and die. It took a long time for her to die, although finally one night, she breathed her last breath. Mrs. Nolan believed it to be a blessing.

When Mrs. Nolan was diagnosed with cancer in the 1990s, memories of her friend flooded back, and she became so anxious she could not function. She knew that pain could be better managed than in Mary's time, but she feared many things: losing control of herself, of bladder and bowel function, of mobility, of the ability to think and to keep her emotions even. Her memories immobilized her so that she could not make a decision about her treatment, refused to see her family, stopped going to church, and began losing weight due to not eating. She could not sleep. At a time when she needed to practice good health habits she gave up exercise and began drinking alcohol to excess.

When a person approaches death, there are two areas of thought that dominate one's time and energy. One combines the apprehension of what is unknown with the desire to avoid what can yet be avoided (like pain). This apprehension is related to fear and anxiety. The other dominant area of thought is bereavement, the anticipatory grieving of the loss of this world and the people one loves (Saunders, 1984, p. 44). Past experience and present knowledge contribute to how a person resolves each of these issues. Grief and bereavement are discussed in chapter 3.

FEAR

People who know they are dying experience a variety of emotions. They can move quickly from one emotion to another. A period of depression and withdrawal may be punctuated by periods of rage and anger. A serene acceptance of the impending death may swing quickly into anxious overactivity and a feeling of panic. Moods may last days and weeks, or minutes. A loving wife may yell at her dying husband, "Why don't you just die right now?" in her frustration of the moment. Any of these emotions in the dying person or the family and friends of that person may be exacerbated by fear. Fear is universal and normal, but not desirable.

Fear and anxiety related to death are sometimes seen in the physical status of the person. Fast heart rate, dry mouth, and quickened respirations are examples of physical cues that stress is overwhelming one's ability to cope. Insomnia and crying are also clues to identification of fear.

There are several specific fears that dying people frequently identify. They can be categorized as fears related to:

- symptoms and potential symptoms
- inability to cope and loss of control
- what comes after death
- changing roles or loss of family and social relationships
- economics and status

There are also several specific fears that health care professionals who care for dying people can identify in themselves. Their fears interfere with communication. They include:

- the inability to do enough for patients (failure)
- fear of expressing emotions in front of others
- fear of blame for poor outcomes
- fear of their own death
- fear of eliciting an emotional reaction in the patient (Buckman, 1993)

Families who care for loved but dying family members experience the same fears as do health care professionals. An old man may not want to go into his wife's room when she is dying because he fears that seeing him weep might make it harder for her. He fears not being able to control his own grief as well as making her feel sad because of his grief. So he denies himself time with her at the end of her life. He may also fear to take her home, not being practiced in the caregiving techniques he believes she needs. If home health care is an option in his community, the simple act of referral may help him to overcome this aspect of his fear.

ANXIETY

Anxiety is different from fear. A mild level of anxiety is useful in that it prods the individual to become alert, watchful, and motivated. A mildly anxious person takes in the information needed to make decisions and take action. But as a person moves from a mild to a moderate anxiety, the alertness changes to preoccupation and restlessness. It is harder to concentrate, and teaching is not as easily accepted. Other mood states, like anger, begin to intrude on the person's thoughts.

Common defense mechanisms like denial may push the anxiety out of mind, but it will reappear. Coping techniques other than defense mechanisms are determined in part by the coping strategies a person has used in the past, by culturally accepted strategies for dealing with death, and by the information and support the patient receives from the health care community and significant support systems.

If the anxiety becomes severe, the patient will experience physiological symptoms, such as tachycardia, increased blood pressure, dry mouth, diaphoresis, insomnia, and trembling. Pacing, irritability, fatigue, and deteriorating relationships are characteristic. The anxiety can progress to a feeling of panic. Mrs. Nolan illustrates what happens when a person approaches severe anxiety. In her case, alcohol abuse and withdrawal were attempts to put the anxiety out of her mind.

Goals of care for Mrs. Nolan and others like her are to use the state of mild anxiety to teach and support the patient, and to intervene appropriately in the stage of moderate anxiety to assist the patient to develop helpful coping strategies. It is important to prevent severe anxiety. Medication is sometimes useful for this, although there are a variety of other treatments that can also be useful.

COPING

Coping is a term describing the behavior one uses to respond to stress. Healthy coping is termed adaptive coping. Maladaptive coping is an unhealthy response to a stressor. Mrs. Nolan's use of alcohol as a behavior triggered by the extreme stress of a diagnosis of cancer and fear of death can be termed maladaptive coping. People develop a pattern for coping throughout life, and they tend to use that pattern (or coping strategy) for any stressor in life. If the pattern is maladaptive, the individual may need help to change it.

Patterns of coping (see table 6.1) may include the use of defense mechanisms defined by Freud. They are used primarily to avoid stress or conflict. For people who are unable to face a fear, especially the fear of death, denial is a defense mechanism that serves the purpose of protecting them from having to deal with the fearful situation. While defense mechanisms are normal and often useful, if prolonged they can be harmful. In denial, for example, several kinds of actions may be delayed or prevented. They include a person's need to act in his own behalf, to take care of problems, and to sustain important relationships. If a person does not pay attention to these things, needed healing for patient and family may not occur.

Sometimes a person may choose to continue a familiar pattern of behavior in the face of new information that should modify the behavior. For example, people who are told that their disease is terminal, and there is nothing the doctors can do, may continue looking for the right doctor, because their pattern for caring for self requires finding the person who can help. They are convinced that the right doctor can help. For an individual who is dying, this may be wasted effort, taking time from more important goals. It is maladaptive behavior.

Thinking clearly in the midst of anxiety, especially anxiety about death, is extremely difficult. Another way to cope is to take

Maladaptive Coping Patterns	Adaptive Coping Patterns
Unconflicted adherence (same behaviors in spite of new information)	Traditional defense mechanisms
Unconflicted change (change in behavior because of advice of another, without self-assessment of the wisdom of the advice)	Vigilance, rational assessment, and action
Hypervigilance or panic	

Adapted from Janis, I., cited in Napholz, 1994, p. 43.

TABLE 6.1   Behavioral Patterns of Coping

anyone's advice or suggestion without thinking it through. Mrs. Nolan might have heard a friend say, "Go have a drink and forget it," thus beginning her maladaptive slide.

A frantic search for answers may be another maladaptive coping behavior. Students who are not prepared for an examination often exhibit excessive anxiety, and try to cram for the exam—wildly searching for right answers instead of learning the information. Their efforts are generally not productive, so are maladaptive.

There are two things to work on to achieve adaptive coping. The first is to work on the relationship between the stressor (in this case, the fear of dying) and the individual. This requires increasing skills in perception (accurate assessment of the stressor and of an individual's strengths) as well as developing skills in intrapersonal and interpersonal communication.

A person who successfully copes with any problem or fear generally confronts the problem and seeks information about it. Problems and fears are discussed with friends and family or health care professionals (Clinch & Shipper, 1993, p. 61). Adaptive coping is seen in the pattern Janis (1982) termed vigilance. An individual follows a rational plan of action that includes assessment of the stressors (including sources of stress other than dying, since a person usually has many stressors in life), a plan of action, and an evaluation of the effectiveness of that action. Mrs. Nolan will achieve vigilance if she can work through her denial, then consider the relative merits of her diagnosis (that is, assess the real risk of death). She will decide what her resources are (including the people she can talk to), what the best treatments are for her under the circumstances, and evaluate that treatment as she goes through it.

This process is not easy, and almost never occurs alone. It is likely that Mrs. Nolan will be working through her problems, then suddenly become so angry at the unfairness of the situation that she wants to throw things. She may have times when she is unable to plan or to talk about her death. Later, she will continue the rational planning, and perhaps work on the relationships between herself and her fears.

The other part of coping is to learn to change some of the psychophysiological results of stress for the individual (Napholz, 1994). Relaxation, humor, imagery, and biofeedback are some techniques people can use to counteract some effects of stress. People have learned to decrease blood pressure, tachycardia, and tachypnia, and increase peripheral blood flow using a variety of techniques. There is some evidence that some people can even improve the functioning of their immune system by using imagery, though not everyone agrees that there is enough evidence to state this as fact.

Not everyone chooses to try to learn to control physiology, especially if they are very ill. They should not be made to feel that they have failed if they cannot control blood pressure, or respiratory rate, or other bodily functions. Like other patterns of coping, the use of these techniques is determined in part by culture and experience. The competent nurse finds the healing methods that work for the patient according to the goals and values of that patient. For many Americans, medication is the treatment of choice.

ASSESSMENT

Ideally, adaptive coping begins with an accurate self-assessment of three things: the situation; the individual's own thoughts and fears related to death; and the other people involved. Individuals perceive situations differently and have fears that interfere with the ability to think clearly. An accurate assessment of the situation is often difficult unless a person can talk with someone who is able to reflect and clarify his perceptions. For example, Sam may become anxious because he believes he is gaining a great amount of weight from the treatments he is taking. After talking with a nurse to clarify his perception, he may decide to keep a record of his weight measured by a scale. This is a rational (logical) approach that will clarify the scope of the problem. Reflecting and clarifying what a patient is perceiving in relation to disease, treatment, and healing is often the task of the nurse. Setting goals, planning how to achieve them and evaluating whether they have been met are mutual processes between the dying person and the nurse (or other caregiver). The nurse is often responsible for the accuracy of the information upon which the patient makes choices. Examining a problem is difficult if it causes an individual to focus on it for long periods, and can lead to more anxiety. Mature coping requires accurate information upon which to develop a plan for action and the determination of end-of-life goals and relationships.

A sick person needs to know physical limits, and psychological and sociological strengths. Accurate assessment includes information about both the stressor and the person's coping skills. A person who has strong coping skills may function quite well in the presence of a very intense stressor, like the diagnosis of a terminal disease. Another person may need a lot of help coping with a small facial scar following the removal of a skin cancer if the coping skills are minimal.

Some stressors that require ongoing assessment for the person who is dying include:

- differences in expectations and goals between patient and family

- increasing communication problems between patient and family and caregivers

- problems in symptom management

- difficulty with anticipatory grief, low self-esteem, or early feelings of wanting to die

- guilt that one has done something to cause the terminal illness (Benoliel, 1991)

If any one of these areas is increasing in intensity, it may foster more fear and less ability to cope. It may take time and effort away from the accomplishment of important end-of-life goals.

COMMUNICATION

"Terminal care is a matter of human relationships . . . the challenge and reward of terminal care arise from the fact that it demands that we use the whole of ourselves to relate to fellow human beings who are in trouble" (Saunders, 1984, p. 62). It is most important to remember this when helping the dying patient who is frightened. There are differences in treating the anxiety of the dying patient and the patient who is anxious in response to other kinds of new experiences. For the anxious person, talking it out (ventilation) is the single most effective treatment. Yet, denial of death is common in American society, and this sometimes makes it hard for the dying patient to be able to talk about it. In addition, the family and other people important in the patient's life may be grieving, and find it difficult to talk about death. Helping a person talk about the immediacy of death in a personal way may be the most important care a health care professional can give. In the talking, healing relationships can be established, continued, or reestablished.

The healing relationship may have begun long before the patient was diagnosed with a life-threatening or life-ending disease, if there is an ongoing relationship with health care professionals—a family doctor, hospice nurses from a previous experience with the death of a loved one, or a nurse on a special unit in the hospital. If not, a conscious effort to establish relationship should begin during the diagnosis phase of the illness. When the physician tells the patient and family of the prognosis, the nurse is usually present and stays with them to offer support after the physician leaves the room. If the family has questions, they can be answered quickly and factually as they arise. It is important to be sensitive to the family, establishing the rapport that will lead to a healing relationship. Ramona's case illustrates the help a nurse can give to a family in limiting the fear and severe anxiety experienced after hearing the news of a family member's impending death.

Ramona and Julio

Ramona entered the hospital for a diagnostic workup, basically feeling good, but with lymphadenopathy. Upon reflection, she remembered that she was more tired than usual, and her appetite was poor. After a series of tests, the doctor and nurse went to discuss Ramona's case with her and her husband, Julio.

Taking time to close the door of the room and sit, the doctor told them that the tests indicated a serious condition, a form of cancer for which there was little that medicine could do. He told them that there was always hope, and that about 10 percent of people with her condition did go into long-term remission. The doctor explained treatment options to a couple who were stunned. He told them he was available to answer questions, but that he would give them some time to think about what he had said. Then the doctor left the room.

Ramona began crying and Julio sat on the bed and held her tightly. The nurse closed the door and waited quietly. They realized she was still there when she handed them tissues. Julio began clenching his fists, and he asked the nurse how the doctor could be so sure of his diagnosis. Should they seek another doctor? For almost 30 minutes Ramona and Julio alternated their statements between "It can't be true—it can't be happening to us," and "There must be some mistake—the laboratory tests were wrong, the doctor doesn't know the latest." The nurse knew there was no answer to those questions, so she remained quiet, alert, and centered. Finally, Julio said, "Ramona can't die. I need her." The nurse said, "This is a time when it seems you need each other." She encouraged them to continue doing what they were doing, talking about how each of them felt and what to do about the future, together. She told them that they had some time, there was no rush. They could plan how best to tell family and friends and what information they needed to make decisions about treatments. She encouraged them to list the questions they had, and to include the hard things, like "How does it feel to die." She left with the promise to return in 30 minutes, sooner if they called.

Recognizing that each time she saw Ramona and/or Julio the interview would be different, the nurse reassessed the situation at each interview, never taking for granted their responses or their knowledge. She focused on helping them learn to confront the situation and get the information they needed to make decisions, and allowing them to discuss their fears and plans. Each contact, though different, was always characterized by presence, caring, and competency by the nurse.

There are a number of useful communication techniques that can be used to develop a helpful relationship like the one between the nurse and Ramona and Julio. The nurse needs to take in all the information that is being offered by those in the relationship. The nurse needs to respond to them.

Taking In Information

Taking in information requires consciously attending to all that is going on at that moment. Paying attention is vital, the most important part of communication, and includes the use of self. The concept of presence, which was discussed earlier, is a part of paying attention. Honesty and a feeling of trust and respect are behaviors that help both people benefit by the interaction. During an interaction, it is necessary to control distractions as much as possible; e.g., by turning off a beeper or a distracting TV. It may not be possible to control all distractions, like the telephone, but fewer interruptions make it easier to pay attention.

There are some physical behaviors that help communication between people. There are very few times, if ever, that a health care professional should give sensitive, possibly devastating information to a patient or try to comfort a patient who has received such news while standing over the person. Standing while a patient is in bed or sitting, and trying to carry on an intense conversation can easily be intimidating and frightening. Some caregivers tend to link a soft voice with empathy. But if the patient cannot hear what is being said, trying to hear becomes a distraction that will not easily be tolerated.

The nurse should sit fairly close to the patient, facing him and leaning slightly toward him at eye level to see and be seen clearly. A summary of helpful behaviors follows.

- Maintain appropriate eye contact.

- Sit close enough to hear well and speak in a normal voice, but not so close that it is distressing for either person.

- Use an open, nondefensive posture to give an indication of the level of involvement.

- Avoid folded arms, rigid stance, or leaning backwards.

- Speak loud enough.

- Use all the senses, and notice if there is a change or difference, such as an odor, or if the person begins to feel cold and clammy. Attending to these sensations may help to validate what the patient is saying.

- Provide privacy and comfort during interviews and interactions.

Active listening is a total effort to grasp the facts and feelings expressed by others. The primary goal is to understand the situation as the other person sees it. Nurses are taught the basics of active listening early in their nursing careers, but emphasis on skill acquisition and information needed to begin a career sometimes means that the nurse gets little practice in really listening to the patient. Listening to the person is the major skill to be developed by the nurse, the area of greatest need for the person who is dying. Fear cannot be alleviated or symptoms controlled unless the patient is heard and the messages about the state of the symptoms or the effect of fear in a life can be assessed. A good active listener is

- fully alert

- oriented to the here and now of the interaction

- interested in the person and what each individual has to say

- tuned in to both verbal and nonverbal communication

- able to suspend own frame of reference

Responding

Taking in information during an interaction with a dying patient is only a part of the communication process. The other part is responding. Three basic but very useful techniques in responding are reflection, clarification, and silence.

Reflection is an accurate paraphrase of the essence of what a person has said. This technique lets the person feel heard and understood, and it does not evaluate the interaction. The paraphrase may include the facts or the feelings or both. For example, when the nurse found Julio in the hallway one evening some months after the initial diagnosis, he said, "My wife is dying. I'm too angry to go in there and see her. I'm tied up in knots inside, and she gets upset if I am upset." The nurse had three choices of responses. She could respond to the facts, the feelings, or both facts and feeling.

Responding to the facts, she might say, "You don't want your wife to see you upset." Responding to feelings, she might say, "You're angry." Responding to both facts and feelings, she might say, "You're angry, and don't want to get upset in front of your wife." Any of these responses are good. The best is probably the one that responds to both fact and feeling, because the person will feel he has been heard, that he is not judged because of his anger, and he can continue talking.

Clarification develops, expands, and amplifies a person's comments. This is a useful technique when the person makes unclear or confusing statements. Clarification starts with a tentative opener like, "It appears that" or, "It sounds like" or "I think I hear you saying that." The nurse might clarify what Julio said by saying something like, "It sounds like you are saying that you feel concerned about your wife, but you think that her seeing your anger about the situation will only make her feel worse. You're afraid of what might happen to her because you are angry." This is helpful if Julio has not sorted out why he feels upset, and allows him to go on talking without being judged for feeling afraid or sounding unsure of himself. This answer also gives him the opportunity to correct any misperception on the part of the nurse.

Silence is a method of communication that allows two people to interact without the use of words. Silence does three things. It tells a person that it is not necessary to entertain the caregiver. The nurse will stay in the room even without conversation if appropriate. Secondly, silence allows both people in the interaction to collect their thoughts. It also encourages the person to continue talking after some time, without embarrassment at a behavior that might be less than appropriate in a social setting.

The rules of communication are guides, not rigid laws. Communicate a sense of wanting to be there. The act of being there, present, attentive, actively listening and responding to need far outweighs any social mistake or slip of the tongue. The expert nurse caring for the dying patient is relaxed in the relationship, knows the goals of a healing relationship, and does not fear saying the wrong thing. The nurse is comfortable with silence and honest with feelings.

SUPPORT GROUPS

Though the nurse can help the patient with expression of feelings leading to improved coping skills, people who are dying are also very effective in establishing healing relationships with each other. Support groups are safe places for people to express feelings they fear others will not understand. The people who are undergoing similar experiences can offer each other understanding, the benefit of experience in practical matters, the knowledge that the group will remember them, and a safe place to be honest when families and others significant in their lives may be disturbed by their fears. In helping each other, each individual finds another meaning to life.

Mary Ann and Roger

Roger needed a heart transplant. His cardiac disease was progressing slowly, his cardiac output decreasing and his fatigue level increasing. It was unlikely he would get a heart in time. A well-qualified clinical nurse specialist had started a support group for people like Roger and his wife. Beginning with an invitation to those people whose names are on the transplant list, the nurse scheduled a time, place in the heart center to meet, and parking vouchers for group members coming to a meeting. Both Roger and Mary Ann were invited. In the 12 weeks that Mary Ann and Roger were a part of the group, they were able to share their constant uncertainty mixed with hope, and their frustrations when Roger's condition began deteriorating significantly and it became clear he would die soon.

When Mary Ann returned to the group after the funeral to say good-bye to the people who had shared such a significant part of her life, they held a brief ceremony to commemorate his life, a kind of healing service. Special things Roger had shared in the group were remembered, and written messages were collected and burned in a small dish, the smoke carrying the messages upward to him. This physical act was a symbolic method of saying good-bye, but Mary Ann was comforted in the knowledge that Roger would be remembered by this group of people.

There are many kinds of support groups. Some are composed of people who are diagnosed with an incurable disease at the same time. More often, a particular institution or group like hospice has one or more support groups available to those who wish to take advantage of them. Some groups are composed of patient and spouse, some include children, some are only for the individual patients. Most groups meet for 45 minutes to an hour, but some groups meet for retreats of a weekend or even a week. Some are focused on specific problems, like anticipatory bereavement. Others are open to any topic. Some have leaders who are professional health care providers. Others are led by the members. Some are even meant to carry on after a person has died, to support the spouse or loved ones.

Camp Bluebird is an example of a special support group for adults with cancer. Not all of those who attend this weekend retreat will die of the disease, but many will. They spend the weekend in a beautiful, natural setting, with individual rooms at a lodge, in the company of each other and volunteers who teach a variety of skills. Some volunteers focus on comfort techniques, allowing the campers to experience massage, Therapeutic Touch, imagery, and meditation. Others focus on self-esteem techniques, like makeovers, choice of wigs, and color and style hints for buying new clothes. Connections with loved ones who are not present are maintained by asking significant people in the campers' lives ahead of time to send a special letter, telling the camper something special about their relationship. The letters are shared as the campers wish, during a time that tends to be quite emotional. Each member of the group builds a bird house, which symbolizes hope. There are several group meetings for ventilation, sharing, and support. Campers return to family, friends, home, or care setting feeling refreshed, renewed, and hopeful. Some of them report a kind of transcendent or spiritual experience.

When starting a support group, several things must be considered. It is helpful to a novice to have the assistance of someone experienced in leading support groups. Competency involves an understanding of group process, the ability to make a clear choice about leadership style (directive versus nondirective, for example), an unambiguous statement about the purpose of the group, and the establishment of membership criteria for the group. For a group of people who may be dying, some understanding of the problems the group members are experiencing may be helpful. For example, if the common problem is increasing loss of control, as in multiple sclerosis, the group will probably share feelings of chronic anxiety more than acute anxiety. The need for specific kinds of information is different in that group from a group waiting for transplants. If the group's purpose is to share feelings rather than get information, the ability to interpret care and treatment plans is less important.

Common needs often addressed in a support group include:

• obtaining guidance

• reassurance of worth

• a sense of reliable alliance among members

• opportunities for nurturance

• attachment

• social integration (adapted from Kinney et al., 1985)

Meeting this set of needs gives the group members additional resources to use in coping with fear and anxiety.

OTHER TECHNIQUES FOR REDUCTION OF FEAR AND ANXIETY

There are several other nursing interventions useful in helping a person control fear and/or anxiety related to dying. Visualization, humor, and life review are three of these techniques.

Visualization

Visualization, seeing something with the mind's eye or making a mental image of something, is a technique often suggested for stress control and healing (Keegan, 1994). Based on the idea that the mind and body are so interconnected that a change in one corresponds in general to a change in the other, people use visualization or specific imagery to decrease feelings of distress. If a person can imagine a scene that makes him feel peaceful, the whole body begins to relax and the signs of anxiety diminish. Anxiety cannot coexist with relaxation. ·

Everyone has had the experience of imagination. It is a universal human phenomenon. People imagine what it is like to receive an award, meet a great person, or win a special competition. Imagining the tart taste of a lemon or the sweetness of cold ice cream makes the mouth water.

Using this natural ability, a person can create a place in the mind that is unique. The created place can contain all the things believed to be necessary for comfort or peace. It is always available and always safe. A skillful nurse can guide the patient in the creation of this place so that it is useful for dealing with the fear related to dying.

When a nurse or someone else guides the creation of an image, the process is termed guided imagery. There are many forms of imagery. The safe-place technique is a process image, an image that can continually be changed as needs change. In guiding the creation of such an image, the nurse builds on several ideas.

- A relaxation exercise is a useful first step when teaching a patient to create the safe place.

- The safe place should be a place that appears soon into the exercise. Do not spend time looking for an ideal image to appear.

- A person can imagine getting to the safe place in a variety of ways, such as taking an elevator up (or down), being carried away by a cloud, or being blown by the wind.

- Indirect suggestions allow the patient to be creative and choose the most comfortable images.

- Daily practice in visiting the safe place helps make it more accessible during particularly stressful times.

- There should be a planned method of reentering the world outside the safe place or image; for example, reversing the steps taken to get into the safe place or exiting the safe place via a slide or another appropriate image.

Mrs. Pond

One dying patient, Mrs. Pond, experienced nightmares involving dying with no one present. She woke up nights in a cold sweat, calling out to her husband and children to hold her hand and stay with her. Before the onset of the nightmares, she had learned to use progressive muscle relaxation for pain control. The nurse suggested she build on that relaxation technique and create a safe place image to help with the anxiety that came after the nightmares. The nurse helped her with a regular progressive relaxation session, and toward the end of it made the indirect suggestion that Mrs. Pond find herself transported across time and space to a place that meant peace and happiness. After a short time of silence, further suggestions were made that Mrs. Pond notice everything in the safe place and remember it so she could return to it later, and that she be transported back to the present feeling refreshed and calm.

Mrs. Pond later reported that during the session she found herself on a sled, being whisked through the air like Santa Claus to a place filled with light, warmth, and soft animals—rabbits, koala bears, and most importantly, a large white cat. The cat immediately curled up on her lap, purring and offering the comfort only animals can give, in this case a very tactile kind of support. The nurse reminded Mrs. Pond that she could return to her safe place during any relaxation session, even after an upsetting nightmare, and recapture the feeling of peace and of being loved. She needed only to become relaxed and call her sled.

Imagery can also be used to rehearse an event about which a person is fearful. It is well-known that prior to chemotherapy some patients become nauseated and even vomit in anticipation of the treatment, almost living the event before it happens. Rehearsing the session of chemotherapy as imagery allows the patient to create more positive outcomes in the images; for example, a session in which no vomiting occurs. The body will often respond to the rehearsed sensations as practiced.

The imagery used to rehearse a situation (surgery, endoscopic examination, medication, and so on) should be based on accurate information. If the procedure is uncomfortable, that fact should be included. It can be related to something coped with successfully in the past, and be given positive meaning. For example, a procedure requiring a needle insertion may be related to a past mosquito bite, with the suggestion that the patient has successfully managed bites before. If a medication burns while being infused into a vein, the image can be one of power and strength of medication being sent to fight disease. Power surging through the body can be transformed into energy, the ability to eat or take fluids, or whatever is realistic in the situation—the positive goal set by patient and nurse together.

It is also possible for the patient to imagine what it feels like to die. Suggesting this to a relaxed patient should only be done by someone experienced in caring for dying patients. It is a useful technique for helping a person cope with the reality of dying, but the caregiver must be able to handle the needs the patient brings up as a result of the session.

Guided imagery is a planned intervention, and it takes some skill to use it effectively. It is not used to run away from problems or avoid dealing with issues. The patient is still given all the information needed to make decisions, and time to talk about problems. Social interactions are still vital. The image of a safe place gives a kind of time out from the intensity of a situation, and can refresh and strengthen a patient so that issues can be addressed calmly.

Humor

Laughter and humor make a person feel good. Even scripture says "a merry heart doeth good like a medicine . . ." (Proverbs 17:22).

Humor helps promote health physically, as in the respiratory effects of a deep laugh; psychologically, as a coping skill; and cognitively, as a distraction. It can turn a negative event into a less intense one. There are few negative effects of humor, though a patient must be made to feel that people are laughing with him, not at him, or a sense of distrust will develop.

The appropriate use of humor begins with caregivers who are able to have fun together. In a creative and open environment, nurses who are able to laugh at themselves and with others are able to communicate more freely and experience less tension in the work setting. That freedom allows the caregiver to laugh at the jokes the patient tells, and in turn, the shared laughter brings the two closer together in the healing relationship.

Other uses of humor include:

- ice breaker
- decrease stress
- cope with emotions
- release anger
- facilitate learning
- promote socialization
- manage a delicate situation
- share vulnerability
- improve communication
- release hostility
- provide distraction
- give reassurance

The ability to tell a funny story may not be everyone's talent. But everyone can laugh, appreciate a good story, and perceive things in the situation as funny, odd, or ironic. Many people can contribute to the development and use of a humor cart, box, or bag. Used in places where patients may have to stay a long time, the humor cart can be a planned nursing intervention for anyone who needs a good laugh. Some items that might be included are funny videotapes, joke books, cartoons, disguise kits, clown noses, hats, rubber spiders, whoopee cushions, plastic food or drink, and anything else people contribute that makes them laugh.

Humor can also indicate that a person is beginning to recover from a tense, stress-filled event. Two brothers and a father stopped in a restaurant after the funeral of a third brother. They had been through an intense confrontation with death and had found support in each other. They had a short time until they would separate and go to their own homes. When the server asked for the predinner drink orders, the responses were: martini-dry; martini-very dry; cola-wet. The server laughed at the "wet," the family began to laugh, and each knew at that moment that the others would be all right and would get through the grief. The joke was small, but the meaning was significant.

Life Review

Life review is a nursing intervention in which a person is led through a remembrance of life, stage by stage. It is a kind of reminiscence that is structured and planned. Life review has been shown to help depressed people and people dealing with end-of-life issues to work toward a sense of integration of life events, a sense that their lives are unique and meaningful (Haight, 1991). When a person at the end of life is anxious due to a sense of meaninglessness and alienation, planned life review may help.

People who have lived through a near-death experience (NDE) often report that during the experience they saw every event in their lives in exactly the same moment. Graduations, weddings, funerals, and every other important event occurred at the same time during the NDE. Interestingly, old people, who tend to reminisce naturally and without help, do not report life review as a part of the NDEs they may have. Some researchers believe that this is evidence for the fact that the life review is such an important psychological task that if a person does not do it beforehand, the person will do it at the moment of death.

Life review can be conducted in a group, but it is more effective individually. The six to eight sessions parallel Erickson's stages of life, from birth to old age. Open-ended questions for each session/stage can be guided by Haight's Life Review and

Experiencing Form (LREF) (see Appendix 2). Each session is about 45 minutes in length. As a person goes through the work of reviewing life events honestly, pain may be felt since part of life has been painful. But toward the end of the sessions, and particularly in a summary session, an individual usually begins to feel a sense of integration with the past and the present, a kind of wholeness to life. This leads, in turn, to greater peace, less unfinished business.

When conducting life review for young people who are dying, not all the stages will be represented. But a life, no matter how long, is still a complete life. Assisting a patient to see life as a whole is a comforting goal.

PSYCHIATRIC ILLNESS IN DYING

While fear and anxiety are common problems for those who are dying, and can often be helped using the techniques and nursing treatments discussed previously, psychiatric disorders are different and require different treatment. Psychiatric disorders may be a problem for some dying people before they acquire the terminal disease, and the fact that they are dying does not alter that. Psychiatric illness may also be stimulated by the illness. Anxiety may become panic, a person in pain may become depressed, a dementia may develop as a result of an organic process found in HIV infection or a brain metastasis. All of these conditions are treatable.

Treatment of psychiatric conditions is necessary to achieve the goal of care for people who are dying: to be alert and aware, able to communicate with loved ones, with symptoms controlled until the time of death. Another reason for starting or continuing psychiatric treatment for people who need it is that the illness may make it difficult to care for them if they are not treated. For example, a person may become hostile and combative because of paranoia associated with organic brain disease. Treatment of the psychiatric problem requires special expertise, and if successful, makes the healing relationship much easier to achieve.

Panic, depression, and dementias are conditions that the nurse should not deal with alone. Since they often require medication and/or psychotherapy, referral to a qualified provider is an appropriate option. If untreated, patients are at risk for insomnia, attempts at suicide, and the inability to form or continue supportive, healing relationships. Resources for psychiatric referrals are listed in table 6.2.

Advanced practice nurses:*

Psychiatric nurse practitioners

Clinical nurse specialists in psychiatric nursing

Psychiatric liaison nurses

Psychiatrists and some medical doctors

Emergency psychiatric services:

Mobile crisis units

Psychiatric liaison teams in hospitals

Hot lines offering referral services for special symptoms, such as threats of suicide

Psychiatric counselors, depending on licensing laws in each state:

Psychologists

Social workers

---

*Some advanced practice nurses have prescriptive privileges, and can offer both counseling and medication.

TABLE 6.2 Resources for Treatment of Psychiatric Illness in Dying Patients

---

SUMMARY

People who are dying often fear the night, the process of death, losing loved ones, and pain and suffering, and become increasingly anxious. Using excellent communication skills, the nurse helps the individual and family to develop coping skills, and works toward developing a healing relationship. Within the healing relationship, patient, family, and nurse have choices about appropriate techniques to use to decrease fear and anxiety, such as support groups, visualization, humor, or life review. The nurse who establishes a healing relationship with a fearful or anxious patient helps that person to live more fully until death occurs.

References

Benoliel, J. (1991). Multiple meanings of death for older persons. In E. M. Baines (Ed.), *Perspectives on gerontological nursing*, Newbury Park, CA: Sage Publications.

Buckman, R. (1993). Communication in palliative care: A practical guide. In D. Doyle, G. W. C. Hanks, & N. MacDonald (Eds.), *Oxford textbook of palliative medicine.* Oxford: Oxford University Press.

Clinch, J. & Shipper, H. (1993). Quality of life assessment in palliative care. In D. Doyle, G. W. C. Hanks, & N. MacDonald (Eds.), *Oxford textbook of palliative medicine.* Oxford: Oxford University Press.

Haight, B. K. (1991). Psychological illness in aging. In E. M. Baines (Ed.), *Perspectives on gerontological nursing.* Newbury Park, CA: Sage Publications.

Janis, I. (1982). *Stress, attitudes and decisions: Selected papers.* New York: Praeger Publishers.

Keegan, L. (1994). *The nurse as healer.* Albany, NY: Delmar Publishers.

Kinney, C. K. D., Mannetter, R., & Carpenter, M. (1985). Support groups. In G.M. Bulachek & J. C. McCloskey, *Nursing interventions: Treatments for nursing diagnoses.* Philadelphia: W.B. Saunders Co.

Napholz, L. (1994). Promoting adaptive responses to stressors. In P. Beare & J. Myers, *Principles and practices of adult health nursing.* St. Louis: C.V. Mosby Co.

Saunders, C. (1984). *The management of terminal malignant disease* (2nd ed.). London: Edward Arnold Publishers, Ltd.

7 | SPIRITUALITY

THE NATURE OF SPIRITUALITY

Bernie Siegel, physician and author, once threatened to form a group of people who would eat only high-fat meals, learn to smoke, become "couch potatoes," and seek little or no exercise. Siegel had talked with so many desperately ill people who had experienced a deeply moving, life-changing spirituality during the struggle to cope with the disease, he decided that his little band would seek to develop a terminal illness so they could experience transcendence! Said in humor, he nevertheless hit upon a profound truth. No one consciously seeks to be sick, but during illness and dying, sometimes a special kind of inner strength is developed.

There are probably as many definitions of spirituality as there are people. Most definitions incorporate the idea that spirituality includes reaching out from one's inner self both horizontally and vertically. The horizontal dimension refers to a connectedness with others, a "nonreligious sense of life purpose and life satisfaction" (Champagne, 1989). The vertical dimension refers to one's relationship with one's god, the Universe, or of something greater than self. It gives a sense of meaning. Both the horizontal and vertical dimensions transcend, or move beyond, the physical world. A healing relationship involves both dimensions. A healing relationship involves spirituality, because it involves connectedness to others, and a sense of meaning.

Reducing the concept of spirituality to definitions is an academic exercise that is necessary to study ways of assisting dying people. But somehow definitions of spirituality never seem to capture the real essence of this most beautiful part of human experience. The spirit of a person is what gives meaning to life, integrates body and mind, and identifies the individual as unique and as having intrinsic value just for existing. It is part of the mystery of life, requiring us to act morally and responsibly to others as well as to search for the Transcendent. Our spirit energizes us and gives us purpose and direction. It makes us whole, unified in all parts of our being. Caring for oneself inescapably involves care of one's spirit.

SPIRITUAL DEVELOPMENT

Westerhoff (1976) believed that spiritual development occurs throughout life, and defined four stages of faith:

- *experienced* faith, occurring in childhood by interaction with others (such as family) of a similar faith tradition
- *affiliative* faith, occurring in late adolescence, developed by actively participating in activities of a faith tradition, such as youth groups, missionary work, meditation groups
- *searching* faith, a part of young adulthood, developed by questioning and searching and doubting one's faith
- *owned* faith, the faith of commitment, a mature faith

In this model, the early stages of spiritual growth, or the acquisition of faith, are more focused on the horizontal relationship with family and friends. This parallels social development. As one matures, the vertical component of spirituality develops.

It is the internal struggle and search for meaning that is so characteristic of young adults that changes the direction of the relationship to a more vertical attribute. One can imagine spiritual development in this stage using the metaphor of a young tree putting roots solidly into the ground. The tree stretches its branches upward, receives warmth from above, and becomes a conduit for the nourishment from the earth to all parts of the tree, and beyond. Like the spiritually mature person, the tree becomes strong, has its own identity, yet is able to support others. The cycle of the seasons, including falling leaves giving way for new buds, suggests continuity of life. Most spiritual traditions include a sense of continuity of life, continuity of the vertical axis of spirituality. While there are many models of spiritual development, Westerhoff's model is useful for its simplicity and parallel structure to psychological development.

It is possible to develop either the horizontal axis of spirituality or the vertical axis, rather than both. One dying patient became intensely interested in writing a family history. He used his last few months to trace the origins of his family through genealogical charts. He found meaning in his own life in a connectedness to those around him, his place on the family tree defined, through exploring the horizontal aspect of his spirituality. Human relationships were his main interest.

In the early centuries of Christianity, groups of monks sought to develop a relationship with God, and understand the mysteries of life in that way. They were called the Desert Fathers. They spent their lives "striving to re-direct every aspect of body, mind and soul to God" (Ward, 1975). For these men, the vertical relationship between themselves and God was all important. This gave their lives meaning. They were hospitable to travelers and shared their meager supplies with anyone in need, but they did it as service to God, not as connection with people.

SPIRITUAL HEALTH

For most people, spiritual health requires the development of spirituality in both the horizontal and vertical directions throughout the life span. It is not static, but a dynamic ebb and flow of energy that helps one to feel satisfied with life. The National Interfaith Coalition on Aging (NICA) defines spiritual well-being in part as the "affirmation of life in a relationship with God, self, community and environment that nurtures and celebrates wholeness" (Cook, 1980).

People who have faced a life-threatening illness and learned to live with it peacefully tell of a journey inward, going into a place within themselves where they learn to accept the fact of the illness. This is not a resignation or defeat. They find a courage that enables them to embrace life as it is now, a kind of inner wisdom. They decide to live before they die, and set realistic goals for today and tomorrow. One man took part in a race he had always wanted to do, another opened a business. A woman decided to live until her first grandchild was born. In some cases the illness went into long-term remission. In others, it did not. But each of the people who adopted this attitude talks of dying as "life enhancing" (Kussman, 1993).

When illness and impending death threaten an individual, the self is always threatened. Death threatens the physical continuity of existence. People search for new meaning and understanding for the whole person at that time. Dr. Elizabeth Kübler-Ross suggested that death does not occur in an instant, but is a continuous process throughout life. Therefore, she suggests that people befriend death, see it as a companion along the path of life. She suggests that befriending death allows one to "truly live your life rather than simply pass through it" (Kübler-Ross, 1975). This distinction refers to depth and meaning in life, a spiritual characteristic. If a person has been able to take the advice of Dr. Kübler-Ross, the threat may be less severe. Denial of death, which is common in American society, interferes with a person's ability to befriend death.

SPIRIT AND MIND

There is a relationship between spiritual and psychological health. Because people function as whole, indivisible beings, anyone who has difficulty in forming relationships due to lack of psychological development or psychological problems may not be able to form relationships in the spiritual sense. Part of spirituality is the ability to love and be loved. Caring for the dying person who has spiritual need and helping that person move toward spiritual health requires caring for that person in the psychological areas of being as well. Excellent communication skills, role-modeling appropriate relationships and connectedness, and establishing trust are mental health skills that are useful in providing spiritual care.

RELIGION AND SPIRITUALITY

Spirituality is a universal human attribute. Everyone is spiritual. Religion is a formal system for the expression of a doctrine or belief. Not everyone has clearly articulated a system of belief, nor joined a religious group. Many people who feel themselves to be spiritual do not admit to being religious. And people who demonstrate an intense religiosity—an outward form of formalized, ritualistic religious behavior, may not appear to be spiritual to others.

Members of many religious groups record a moment of spirituality, perhaps a transcendent moment in a piece of great art, literature, or music, enriching life for all who see or hear it. Stained glass windows, Tibetan chimes, Christmas cantatas, and chants from a variety of religious traditions are examples. Individuals also record their spiritual depths in great art of all forms. Michelangelo's Pieta and Sufi poetry have the power to move, to reach the inner soul. Those present at a performance or in an artistic milieu resonate together, creating a special bond that helps each one to identify meaning in life from the aesthetic ambience that the authors, artists, or composers created.

Formal religious affiliation serves as an expression of spirituality. It can be a kind of spiritual support group. Shared rituals and rites, and transmission of values through the generations nurture and provide benchmarks of an individual's journey through life. They help establish belongingness and love. The wedding ceremony and funeral services are two examples. Those members of a religious faith who are absent from a planned group meeting or service may feel they are sustained in the memory of the group, and perhaps by prayer. Those who are near death may take comfort in the thought that they will be remembered, both by family and friends, and by their deity.

However, there can be problems within an organized group. Any formally constituted group of people, including church, synagogue, or mosque, has expectations of its members. These expectations may conflict with the way an individual feels. If members of an organized religion believe that death is reunion with God, or a doorway to a new life, and should be viewed as a positive event, the anxiety a dying person feels may be seen as failure to live up to expectations. If that occurs, the patient may choose not to use the group for support, diminishing a useful resource for reducing anxiety and moving toward wholeness. Clergy can be very helpful in assisting the patient to understand that anxiety and fear are normal, that spirituality does not depend upon a certain feeling about one event, and that the organization and God are not synonymous. The perceptive nurse exercises tact and a special sensitivity with both the clergy and the patient when there is conflict or guilt because of feelings of failure to live up to a perceived standard of behavior. In this case, the consultation with the clergy should include (with the patient's permission) the fact of the patient's anxiety about the need for dialogue between them. A working relationship and mutual respect between health care providers and clergy in the community helps the consultation process.

Some groups have a statement of belief, hold to a commonly accepted statement of values, and invoke a higher power but do not identify themselves as religious organizations. Alcoholics Anonymous and other 12-step self-help programs are examples of such groups because they have expectations and rites based on values and a belief in a higher power, which some equate with religion. Group membership is one form of spirituality, and provides the support needed to grow toward health.

If a person who is dying has expressed spirituality within a religious group, the group may be an important support during the time of dying. Religion as an expression of one's spirituality is a great help to many people, even if they have been away from it for some time.

Mr. Bower and the Priest

It was clear that Mr. Bower had a question. He waited for several hours for Ms. F., who was busy that night. He smoked in the lounge, dozed in a chair in his room, and walked the hall. When the nurse sat down, he called to her and suggested she "take a break" and sit in the day room with him for a few minutes. Recognizing his need to talk, she did so. His question took a few minutes to be asked, but it was simple. "I haven't been to church for 15 years. I used to be Catholic. Would it be fair to call the priest just because I'm dying?" At 3:00 A.M. in a darkened solarium with a lonely man nearing the end of his life, Ms. F. identified the problem as another relationship that needed healing. He discussed his problem of whether to call the priest or not for two weeks. He was not sure it was fair to God, fair to the church, or fair to himself to reopen his connection with formalized religion. After exploring what it meant to him to be fair, he recognized that it was OK to do something for himself based on his own idea of need. Men have needs, too, even veteran military men who have been self-sufficient for most of their lives. The priest was called. Mr. Bower began to work on his relationship with God, and his priest helped him.

SPIRITUAL NEED AND SPIRITUAL DISTRESS

Spiritual need has been defined as "any factors necessary to establish and/or maintain a person's dynamic personal relationship with God (as defined by that individual) and out of that relationship to experience forgiveness, love, hope, trust and meaning and purpose in life" (Stallwood & Stoll, 1975, p. 1088). The North American Nursing Diagnosis Association (1994, p. 49) calls *spiritual distress* "a state in which an individual experiences a disruption in the life principle which pervades a person's entire being and which integrates and transcends one's biological and psychosocial nature." These definitions are useful in the assessment of spiritual needs and the provision of nursing care. They suggest that forgiveness, love, hope, trust, and meaning and purpose in life are necessary to limit disruption in the integrating and transcending force in a person's life. The definitions also suggest that those characteristics are present as a result of a relationship with God (as defined by that individual). The nurse may discover that the key to helping a person in spiritual distress is to find ways to help preserve and restore those qualities, and support an individual's relationship with the divine.

Forgiveness

Mr. Bower wanted to reestablish a connection with his former religious affiliation, but before he could do so, he needed to experience forgiveness. His separation from his church only began to be a problem that he identified toward the end of his life. The reasons for the separation did not really matter. He harbored no anger or memories that made the reunion fearful or awkward. He simply wanted to return. The separation had begun to interfere with his relationship with God. His fear was that others would judge him, or consider him unworthy. Perhaps God would, as well. He felt guilty. A formal reconciliation and reaffirmation of faith was helpful to him.

Spiritual forgiveness is not always a matter of going back to a group. Some people need to be forgiven by their God figure, for a previous wrong (sin); by other people they believe they have wronged; or by themselves. The experience of Joe and Debbi illustrates the point.

Joe and Debbi

Joe and Debbi believed that God had answered their prayers when their young daughter, who had been diagnosed with leukemia, went into remission. When she relapsed and subsequently died, Joe and Debbi lost their faith. They felt betrayed by God who had reneged on a promise. They stopped attending church and denied God's existence. In their anger, they said things to friends about God that they later felt guilty about. Their anger and guilt made reconciliation difficult, because they found it hard to forgive themselves for what they had felt and said. Guilt and anger are often signs of the need for forgiveness and spiritual reconciliation.

Hope

Hope is a vital spiritual need. Hope is the willingness to embrace all of life's possibilities. Siegel (1986) suggested that hope is energy, that lack of hope is a wish to die. In this context, the wish to die is not a peaceful letting go of life with tasks completed and planned entry into the mystery of death, but a giving up because it is too hard to live. Hope means that there is a future. Hope is correlated with a feeling of well-being. A general kind of hope for the best life possible under the conditions is as useful as hope that has a more defined goal.

Hope may be specific or nonspecific. Specific things to hope for include:

- some new treatment or drug to prolong life
- physical restoration
- the ability to love and be loved
- reconciliation with something or someone in the past
- finding meaning in the mystery of death (Speck, 1993)

Health care providers who tell the patient there is nothing more that can be done interfere with hope. There is always something that can be done in a caring relationship, even if it is only the provision of comfort and relief of pain. Dr. C. Northrup (Kussman, 1993) always tells her patients who have a poor diagnosis/prognosis of the four or five miracles in her patient population, the people who were supposed to die of a disease and did not. It is not ethical to promise cure or anything else that can't be delivered, but it is useful to tell the truth—that some people do live in spite of poor odds. No one knows why. There is hope. This is not to be confused with denial, a refusal to see the possibility of one's death, or to see the signs and do the things necessary to care for one's self given the circumstances present. Hope in this context is to see all the possibilities, including that of life.

There are many things that can interfere with hope. A long parade of strangers who go into and out of a room without really seeing the patient, as in rounds by students from a variety of health care disciplines, may inadvertently give the message that the patient doesn't count any more. People feel that because cure is not foreseen, their case is hopeless but curious. Taking the time to make sure the patient is included in the discussion, and asking about plans and goals for today, give hope. Patients should be partners in the healing process, encouraged to make choices about how to live life now. This is also true for the person at home. If the sick room is entered only when it is time to bring a meal, give a medication or treatment, or other care of some kind, the person becomes isolated, feels like a burden, and becomes hopeless. Family, friends, and other support people need to help the person plan, share thoughts and insights, and hope.

Pity also diminishes hope. It is belittling. The person who pities another doesn't see that person in the fullness of who she is. Only the disease or disability is seen. Patients ought to systematically decrease their contact with people who pity them or otherwise bring them down (Kussman, 1993).

Mr. Kashu (see chapter 2) gave up hope when he felt betrayed by his son. When family relationships are strained and not working, loss of hope can be the result. All the things done to support family relationships while a person is close to death assist to maintain hope.

Trust

People who feel abandoned at a critical time get angry. If the illness that is likely to end in death is the reason for the anger, the angry behavior may be aimed at the nurse. The same techniques for handling anger in other settings are useful, including helping the patient to identify the anger and the reason for the anger; setting appropriate limits on destructive behavior; and, most importantly, using honesty, presence, and genuine caring to help develop a sense of trust. Trust is like the support for the bridge of reconciliation that allows an individual to move from a land of isolation, anger, guilt, and fear to a land where relationships, love, hope, and meaning can exist.

The ability to trust is learned early in life, and if it is not, an individual probably has had difficulty with relationships throughout life. A history of having had at least a few long lasting relationships in life is helpful information in assessing a patient's ability to trust in the present time. A person who feels abandoned and who is no longer able to trust others feels powerless, empty, afraid, and possibly out of control. The nurse who gives the patient reason to trust by providing clear and accurate information, appropriate reassurance, and some control over the treatment process is giving spiritual care.

Meaning

Frankl (1952) suggested other characteristics of spirituality that can be lived within a group or individually. Three areas of values that give meaning to people who are suffering are the opportunity to create or achieve tasks; the ability to experience goodness, truth, beauty, or a significant relationship; and the choice of attitude a person takes toward the suffering. Frankl studied spirituality in relation to survival of concentration camp experience during World War II. Survivors of the camps were the people who could find a weed along the road and see beauty in it, remember a spouse with great tenderness, and even laugh at how they were beginning to smell when the soap ran out. The attitude that led to making a joke of tragedy seems to be life-saving. It certainly helps one to experience life more fully.

Neither spirituality nor its expression through religion means that people will remain healthy or avoid suffering. Saints and sinners alike suffer and die. Dossey (1993, p. 34) warned against healers who recommend specific techniques to "transform one's personality, relationships, goals, thought habits, philosophy, and overall orientation to life" in order to achieve certain specific results. No one has shown that terminal illness is a result of imperfection in the way a person thinks, or that if a person can straighten out grievances against others and learn to love or relate to others in a different way, the disease will miraculously disappear. Changing one's relationships and becoming more open should be things a person chooses to do for the sake of the relationship, to meet the felt need of connecting with others so that life is more satisfying now, not for the purpose of avoiding or curing suffering or illness.

Spirituality is not something sought, but something that is. Behaviors and attitudes are manifestations of the spiritual life. Vietnamese Buddhist Priest Thich Nhat Hanh writes of suffering during the worst days of the war. "In that intense suffering, you feel a kind of relief and joy within yourself, because you know that you are an instrument of compassion. Understanding such intense suffering and realizing compassion in the midst of it, you become a joyful person, even if your life is very hard." (Hanh, 1991, p. 125). One can imagine that this gentle monk lived in all three of the areas that Frankl said gave meaning in suffering. He had tasks to do as a result of his compassion; saw goodness, truth, and relationship where he was; and cultivated an attitude of peace in the face of suffering.

SPIRITUAL ASSESSMENT

It is not easy to assess a person's spiritual health or spiritual distress. The interrelationship of psychological and spiritual behaviors like anger mean that assessment of one gives insight into the other. Stoll (1979) listed four specific areas of assessment of spiritual concerns:

- one's concept of God or deity
- source of strength and hope
- significance of religious practices and rituals
- perceived relationship of spiritual beliefs and state of health

During an interview, each of these areas can be assessed using direct questions. Simple questions asking if a god figure or religion is important in a person's life, what one's concept of the deity is, or if prayer is useful help develop insights about that person's spiritual focus. Knowing what things or people gave spiritual strength in the past, what religious practices and rituals give comfort now, and how each of those things affects the person's perceived state of health can form the basis of a plan to assure continued spiritual care based on a person's own choices.

Even without a formal interview, patients can suggest that they are experiencing some degree of spiritual distress. If they talk about a diety or other spiritual topics, even in a lighthearted fashion, this may reveal the fact that much thought is going on regarding their relationship to their own spirituality or faith. Comments about religious functions a patient cannot attend, negative results of prayer, or rejection of clergy all may indicate spiritual distress.

Nonverbal behaviors also may indicate spiritual distress. Some of those behaviors reflect concurrent psychological and physical distress, since a sad spirit results in a distressed person. These are some behaviors that may indicate spiritual distress:

- expressions of anger (toward God or others)
- sleep disturbances
- increased discomfort in the absence of obvious cause
- inconsistent mood (crying, withdrawal, anxiety)
- restlessness
- social isolation
- gallows humor
- preoccupation with questions about meaning of life, God, or suffering
- rejection of people from one's spiritual heritage or background (Carson, 1989)

Assessment of the environment also aids in the plan for spiritual care. There may be religious books, medals, icons, get-well cards with a religious motif, or music that family or friends have brought to comfort a person. A very restless, semicomatose dying man visibly relaxed when a family member played a tape of the music performed at the service the last Saturday the man had been present at his synagogue. That kind of observation is helpful in planning care. However, the nurse must be careful not to overinterpret symbols or behaviors without asking the patient. A book on prayer may be present as a well-meant gift from a friend that the patient has no intention of reading, and no interest in. The fact that the patient has a friend who sends such a book may be more important.

NURSING INTERVENTIONS

Nowhere is the need for healing relationships more important than for the person in spiritual distress. The goal of care for the person in spiritual distress is to assist that person to experience forgiveness, love, trust, hope, and a sense of meaning and purpose in life, based on a dynamic relationship with God (as that person identifies the relationship).

The Nurse

For a nurse who undertakes to help a person in spiritual distress, Carson (1989, p. 21) has some good advice. "Each nurse needs to acknowledge his or her own personal spiritual journey, for it is in the continuous meeting of one's own spiritual needs that one will know the meaning of spiritual well-being. The greatest gift the nurse has to give to clients is one's personal, living, spiritual richness. This gift of one's true self given in care to the client experiencing crisis will inevitably encourage the client toward spiritual well-being."

The nurse's own spirituality will be reflected in the choice of interventions selected. The interventions selected will be based in part on skills discussed in previous chapters, like the communication skills of active listening, reflection, and clarification, or presence, the sense of being fully focused in this moment for this individual. In addition, the nurse who feels secure in spiritual matters may demonstrate a sense of empathy, humility, and commitment.

Empathy requires that one is able to feel in some degree what the patient is feeling, and to be able to put it into words, so that it can be examined by the person. No one feels exactly as another person does, so it is inaccurate to say, "I know how you feel." But a nurse may be able to say, "I'd probably be angry, too, if I were dying before I felt like I was ready. Let's discuss some things we might do that would help you feel better, to get ready." From this discussion, it might be possible to determine resources and strengths the patient might use and relationships to call upon that would alleviate some of the distress.

Humility allows both the client and the nurse to accept each other as finite human beings who don't know all the answers (Carson, 1989, p. 168). The nurse is fully competent in nursing care and able to provide comfort, pain control, and appropriate treatments, but the choices of direction in the client's life, including the meaning of that life, are determined by the client. The nurse simply provides opportunity, environment, and support as needed so that the spiritual journey can be experienced. Commitment is the choice to share the journey with the client for a little while. It means to make one's self available when a patient needs support, even when it is hard to do so. It is often hard to maintain a relationship with a patient through a terminal illness and be present when that person dies. To be committed to sharing this experience with a patient requires that the nurse maintain a healthy spirituality and support system. Chapter 11 gives suggestions for helping nurses and other caregivers maintain their own health in situations that require a great deal of love and giving of self.

Spiritual Help for the Dying

There are at least five very specific things that can be helpful for the spiritual care of the person who is dying. They include: prayer; presence of loved ones; a time to share; assisting the person to finish any business or things still to be accomplished; and giving permission to die.

Prayer and meditation may be a part of religious experience that some people would like to share. For the person who meditates regularly, provision for a period of time without interruption and perhaps for some physical support to help the person maintain his regular meditative position (like sitting in a particular posture) are indicated. For those who pray, a loved one, clergy, or the nurse may choose to share prayer, if it would be comforting. Provision for quiet and privacy should be made. It may be helpful to agree beforehand on the kind of prayer or meditation, so both people involved are comfortable with the arrangements. Prayer can take many forms, so it is important to ask the person about what is comfortable. A familiar prayer that holds special significance or is offered at a particular time may be comforting. For example, a child may be comforted and feel connected with home and family as well as God if assisted to continue a traditional family prayer such as "Now I lay me down to sleep, I pray the Lord my soul to keep; if I should die before I wake, I pray the Lord my soul to take." Prayer and meditation assist a person to maintain trust in something beyond self, a spiritual relationship.

Dossey calls prayer "nonlocal healing" in some instances, pointing out that many studies have shown that even when a person does not know she is being prayed for, the person being prayed for may feel better. Nonspecific prayers, such as "Thy will be done," may be more effective than goal-oriented prayer for a specified outcome (Dossey, 1993). He also makes a clear and well-documented case for the fact that prayer helps. Carson (1989, p. 169) says that through prayer "the individual communicates needs, feelings, fears, love, adoration, and awe to the Creator. In return, God graces the person with a sense of his presence and his abiding love."

The presence of people significant in one's life is important for spiritual well-being. The nature of one's healing relationship with one's own diety or spirituality, including the sense of forgiveness, love, and meaning, is reflected in one's relationship with significant people in life. Limiting visiting hours, especially at the time close to death, is not helpful unless there is a clear reason for it for the patient's well-being. There are many stories, some well-documented, of a loved one appearing at the bedside of a patient in the moments just before death. The loved one seemed to know that death was near, even without having been called to the bedside. The connection between the two people was maintained even at a distance.

People need private time to share. If they participate in rites, such as sacraments or special observances, the time and place should be respected. A visit to the outside of the building may be necessary to see the sun or feel the breeze. This sometimes is a spiritual experience for the person who finds spirituality in a connection with nature. The person with whom the patient shares this experience, a sibling, parent, spouse, or friend, should be encouraged and assisted. The nurse advocates for the patient's right to maintain spiritual connectedness in any way that is useful to the patient and does not interfere with the rights of others.

Grandpa John

Grandpa John was dying, and the end was near. His breathing was labored, and he appeared to be waiting. His family had been called to come to the hospital. The student nurse was sitting at the bedside. Looking out of the window, he saw the old man's family drive up in their battered, well-used car. He told Grandpa John that the family was here. The man looked at the student, smiled, closed his eyes, took one last breath, and died. The student told the family their grandpa had waited for them, and he knew the family had come. That news was comforting to the family. The old man had waited until he had done all he could for his loved ones. Grandpa John had waited to die until his family had come to the hospital, and the fact of their presence gave him permission to die.

Many people seem to wait for permission to die. A child dying of a long-term genetic disease had talked of going to be with God. But on the day that he was so close to death that he was struggling for every breath, he did not die until his mother told him, "I think it is time for you to be with God." His struggles ceased, he was comforted, and he died later that day. His mother had given him peace by giving him permission to die.

SUMMARY

During the course of dying, some people turn toward an inner wisdom that helps them transform the experience from fear, anger, loss, or sense of catastrophe to an ability to embrace all of life. The relationships with family and loved ones deepen and are characterized by forgiveness, trust, love, and an abiding sense of satisfaction and purpose that has been fulfilled. They feel the presence of their God, the universal, the meaning beyond self. Sometimes the nurse is privileged to support the patient through these changes. Providing an environment and resources to allow a person to pursue spiritual development is a part of spiritual care. Assessing for spiritual distress and becoming an avenue of communication in order to support relationships are critical in the relief of spiritual distress and in helping the dying person choose to live fully in the remaining time.

However, the nurse who shares the experience with the patient, who gives of self in presence, humility, empathy, and commitment, shares the satisfaction of a mature spirituality. The nurse cares for self while caring for the patient, and grows in grace and the comfort of healing relationships.

References

Carson, V. (1989). *Spiritual dimensions of nursing practice.* Philadelphia: W.B. Saunders.

Champagne, K. (1989). Value-belief pattern. In G. McFarland & E. McFarland, *Nursing diagnosis & prevention: Planning for patient care.* St. Louis: C.V. Mosby Co.

Cook, T. C. (1980). Preface. In J. A. Thorson & T. C. Cook (Eds.), *Spiritual well-being of the elderly.* Springfield, IL: Charles C. Thomas.

Dossey, L. (1993). *Healing words.* San Francisco: Harper Colliers, Publishers.

Frankl, V. (1952). *The doctor and the soul.* New York: Bantam Books.

Hanh, T. (1991). *Peace is every step.* New York: Bantam Books.

Kübler-Ross, E. (1975). *Death: The final stage of growth.* Englewood Cliffs, NJ: Prentiss-Hall.

Kussman, L. (Producer) (1993). *Harbor of hope.* [Videotape] (Available from Aquarius Productions, Inc., 35 Main St., Wayland, MA 01778)

North American Nursing Diagnosis Association. (1994). *Taxonomy I* (rev. 1990). St. Louis. MO: NANDA.

Siegel, B. (1986). *Love, medicine, and miracles.* New York: Harper & Row.

Speck, P. (1993). Spiritual issues in palliative care. In D. Doyle, G. W. C. Hanks & N. MacDonald (Eds.), *Oxford textbook of palliative medicine.* Oxford: Oxford University Press.

Stallwood, J. & Stoll, R. (1975). Spiritual dimensions of nursing practice. In I. L. Beland & H. Y. Passos (Eds.), *Clinical Nursing* (3rd ed.). New York: McMillan.

Stoll, R. (1979). Guidelines for spiritual assessment. *American Journal of Nursing, 9*: 1574.

Ward, B. (1975). *The sayings of the desert fathers.* Kalamazoo, MI: Cistercian Publications.

Westerhoff, J. (1976). *Will our children have faith?* New York: Seabury Press.

3 HELP FOR FAMILIES

8 | FAMILIES

GOALS

Families provide the primary social support for many sick people. Resources in terms of care, transportation, activities of daily living, and social interaction generally start with the family. But not all families are prepared to provide this support.

Mrs. Peterson

Mrs. Peterson clearly had difficulty moving around, but she told the hospice nurse that she tried not to call her family for help unless she really had to. She had her own bedroom in the eight-room home that was neat and well-kept. There was a television with remote control and a variety of care aids, including the hospital bed in which she slept. Several times during the assessment visit, Mrs. Gage, the hospice nurse, noted family members in the hall passing the bedroom door. They never said anything or even appeared to look into the room.

One young son, a teenager, brought lemonade about 30 minutes into the visit, but did not stay. Mrs. Peterson excused the behavior, saying they were busy and did not have much time to stop and talk. When the nurse asked her why they had waited until so late in the course of her illness to contact hospice, Mrs. Peterson said that they had been managing, and the eldest son who did not live in the home was opposed to hospice. It had taken him until now to permit the call.

Mrs. Gage assessed the situation. Mrs. Peterson was effectively isolated, socially unavailable. Her family provided for physical needs, medications, and entertainment opportunities. They would provide a videotape for entertainment, but would not stay with her to watch it. They seemed uncomfortable around her. When they were not in the home, her friends could not get into the house, so they stopped dropping by. She did some visiting by telephone. The family members meant well, but they led busy lives, and did not recognize that they had a limited time with the wife and mother. They were not dealing with their own feelings about the situation. Talking with the elder son, a professional man who happened to come into the house at the end of the visit, Mrs. Gage asked him why he had been opposed to hospice care. He frankly answered that calling hospice meant that they had given up, that his mother would die. It seemed that by avoiding the call they would avoid the death.

Mrs. Peterson's family met her physical needs for nutrition, hygiene, pain control, and safety. But she was not emotionally connected to the people around her who had given her life meaning. Mrs. Peterson had been the kind of Mom who baked cookies, went to the PTA, and served as room mother for each of her three children's fourth-grade classes. She had entertained her husband's clients and was on the board of the local recreation department. In this final illness, it seemed she was still serving others by not bothering them, which was her long-time pattern of behavior.

Mrs. Gage knew that this was a family in trouble. Unless healing occurred, unless family members and Mrs. Peterson could begin to talk about the future, the family would probably have difficulty grieving later, perhaps experiencing guilt, tension, and prolonged grief. Mrs. Peterson would not be assured of her impact on the lives of others, or of her place in their memories. She might not have the opportunity to say good-bye, to release them from a continued sense of obligation ("I should have done more"), or to do some of the practical tasks for the family that make life easier after the death of a loved one. This family needed help to share the truth of the impending death and what it would mean to them all. If they could share the truth, tension in the home would decrease and a sense of completion of the relationship might be achieved.

Goals of the health care team in this circumstance include:

1. Maintain and support the physical care being given.

2. Increase the numbers of visits to the room for social reasons by helping the family find ways to visit or let friends into the house on a regular schedule.

3. Help the family to begin to talk about Mrs. Peterson's death and its meaning for them.

4. Help Mrs. Peterson to remain connected to her family in spite of their reluctance to discuss serious issues.

5. Make sure Mrs. Peterson has the opportunity to plan for her own future through advance directives, wills, and other legal needs.

CONNECTING

Emotional cutoff (remaining emotionally distant or being unwilling to maintain a relationship at an emotional level) may be both the reason and the result of the inability of the family to talk with each other about an impending death. Generally, as tension in the home (or place where the dying person and family meet) increases, anxiety increases. This leads to deteriorating relationships, explosive outbursts or withdrawal, poor choices and lack of planning for care (especially of self), and eventually a hopelessness and/or depression. Chapter 6 gives some useful techniques for helping people to deal with anxiety.

Long-term illness complicates relationships. If people do not discuss feelings, it seems that everyone involved is living a lie, enacting a sham existence. A patient who may wish for such things as reconciliation with an estranged child, a divorced mate, or an old classmate cannot have them because "the family would not understand" and the topic is taboo. Everyone is protecting everyone else from the truth because the truth hurts, but the results of not living in the truth are separation, isolation, emotional pain, and lack of resolution of the problems. Protecting another from bad news is paternalism.

When a nurse meets a patient who has a suspected terminal diagnosis, it is important to recognize two components of the healing role. The nurse is a role model in truth telling and a patient advocate with the family, the health care team, the institution, and society. This role does not pit the nurse and patient against everyone else. It is likely that everyone involved wants the best for the patient. Creating opportunities for open communication (but not forcing it) will help the group and the patient achieve the best, whatever that is determined to be.

Truth Telling

The Peterson family needed to begin telling each other (and themselves) the truth about why they walk by Mrs. Peterson's room without calling out a hello or dropping in to visit now and then. Mrs. Peterson needed to be able to tell them that she would like them to visit more often, and perhaps share some entertainment or just talk. After beginning to share a few moments, they needed to acknowledge the fact that Mrs. Peterson was dying and some plans had to be made.

Mrs. Gage made a start in helping the family to talk when she asked the son why they called hospice so late. He was able to give an honest and perceptive answer. Many families are not able to admit that death within a defined period of time is probable. This son is moving beyond that stage. Other than denial, reasons why families may not be able to share the truth of an impending death with each other include:

- They have a long history of being unable to share with each other about most things.

- They fear the truth will upset the patient.
- They have insufficient information and do not understand that death is even a possibility.
- Their own feelings about death cause them great anxiety.

A family that has a long history of not sharing with each other, that simply has never communicated, is a challenge for the nurse. It is never easy to break a pattern, but during this most important time in people's lives, there may be an opening that can create new patterns of relationships that are more whole and healthy than previous patterns. This can become a kind of legacy from the one who dies to those who remain in a deeper relationship. Mr. Bower was one who had that experience. Professional counseling is often required to achieve this, and referrals aimed at improving a dysfunctional family's communication patterns should be available to the dying patient and family, just as it is to others.

Mr. Bower Had a Daughter

There was no record of a family for Mr. Bower. He considered his veteran friends his family. It was assumed that he spent his weekend passes with a distant relative, perhaps a cousin or uncle. So when he told Ms. F. about his estranged daughter, she was surprised. By the time he brought it up, he was quite ill. He was ambulatory, but needed regular pain medication in increasing doses, and he tired easily during routine activities like the morning bath ritual.

He had not talked with his daughter for 20 years, but he had gotten her address and wanted to make contact. He was afraid to do so, afraid of rejection. In his post-war years, he had become a heavy drinker and had abandoned his wife and young daughter. He didn't believe that deathbed reunions had fairy tale endings with everyone experiencing a bittersweet reconciliation, and living happily ever after.

But in his search for meaning, he had come to believe that he had done one significant thing in his life, and that was to serve his country during the war. Now he wanted to share that one good thing with his daughter by leaving his medals to her after he died. He wanted Ms. F. to tell him how to do it. Should he call his daughter and tell her what was happening, and risk her refusal to accept his precious gift, the meaning of his life? Should he just have them sent after he died, hoping that she would appreciate them? Was there a course of action between these two roads? Should he just leave his medals to his American Legion Post, and forget the long latent hope of reconciliation?

Ms. F. knew that Mr. Bower had developed good coping skills, and that although rejection by the daughter would be painful, he could cope if he had support. She encouraged him to talk with the staff psychologist to plan the phone call, and promised to be available after he called his daughter. As he had expected, there was to be no joyous reunion. The daughter chose not to visit, but she did appreciate the effort he had made to locate her, and was gracious about the medals, promising to pass them on to the grandson Mr. Bower had never met. Mr. Bower was happy he had called, and the two talked twice more before he died. He knew he would be remembered in the next generation. It was enough.

In some cultures, particularly in the Orient, not telling the patient the diagnosis and poor prognosis is expected behavior. The health care community and the society from which it comes believe that it is useful to protect the patient from potentially devastating news because it may lead to hopelessness and loss of the will to live. But in the United States, Kübler-Ross (1969) wrote of many cases that indicate that the dying patient can handle the "awesome truth" when it is delivered with sensitivity, warmth, and directness. The awesome truth includes how loved ones will be affected, how one is likely to die, and all the other questions to which a person needs an answer. Protecting a person has more to do with rapport, communication skills, the ability to demonstrate caring, and timing than it does with the message (Livingston & Williamson, 1985). Only when the truth is shared does the family realize that the time available for saying "I love you" is limited.

Telling the truth includes giving as much information as the patient and family want, when they want it. Postponing information should only be done when it is clear in the professional judgment of the nurse based on sound patient assessment that the information will be damaging. For example, the nurse will call a team meeting or consult with a physician if an AIDS patient confides that when T-lymphocyte counts reach 200, he plans to commit suicide, and the new results now reflect those levels. The patient will still be told what the results are, but with caution and by the person best able to handle the consequences of the information. Truth in this case would include the fact that the patient had mentioned suicide before, and the nurse wants to know if it is still being considered. The patient may be surprised to still feel reasonably well at this stage, and find there is no reason to end life now. There are still goals to be accomplished. Conversely, the patient may still be considering suicide, and in asking about it, the nurse can initiate helpful interventions, like getting a commitment from the patient not to do anything about suicide until he can talk with the psychiatric liaison nurse or the staff psychiatrist or psychologist.

When truth and honesty are shared, the dying patient may have a change in attitude about the meaning of life and what to do with the time left. It is no longer necessary to spend time and energy being concerned about loved ones, what they might be thinking, things that must be avoided in conversation, what will happen after the death occurs. Loved ones can also plan, know where to go for help (support groups, memorial services, Make-a-wish Foundation, and so on), and say what they want to say now.

Sometimes it happens that the family never feels comfortable enough to share feelings with the dying person before the death. But the sick individual wants to say good-bye, and to leave other messages. These kinds of wishes can be fulfilled with creative use of communications skills and a little planning. A lawyer can help with family financial planning, and write a will that includes special bequests to special people. A tape recorder can be used to record thoughts and messages to be heard after the death, or kept for years until small children reach a certain age and messages are meaningful. A diary of a grandmother included several years of day-by-day routine. It was a great comfort to the family later to realize how many friends had called, how often people shoveled the snow from her sidewalk or ran errands while the family felt guilty for not being there more often. After reading the diary, they knew she led a rich and full life, loved them and the things they accomplished, and had realized that those accomplishments could only occur in the distant city in which the children and grandchildren lived. Through the diary, she absolved them of guilt, a great gift.

The terminally ill patient and family need the truth from each other and from health care professionals. The truth shared compassionately and realistically does several things. It

- decreases anxiety for patient and family

- demonstrates respect and promotes rapport

- provides information for everyone involved

- allows the patient to make decisions for self-care

- provides time for planning

- gives time for the family to gather support

- gives time to achieve resolution of end of life issues

The same results of truth telling are experienced by groups of people who relate to each other around a social issue they work on together, or an intellectual interest, or other common bond. A well-known and much beloved nurse theorist, Dr. Martha Rogers, understood the importance of dealing with death honestly and openly. She had a date to speak to a conference which bore her name—the Rogerian Society. But she also knew she was dying and was not sure she would get to the conference. She did die before the conference, but she had made a tape to play for those gathered there. She used it to say good-bye to many people who had followed her work and admired her greatly. When it was played, it was a moving moment, allowing those present to celebrate the woman and support each other in their loss.

Advocacy

While there are many definitions of patient advocacy, they all include two components. Advocacy involves giving relevant information, and supporting the decisions made by the patient. Advocacy is based on the moral right of people to self-determination. Two of the three characteristics Gadow (1980) used to describe advocacy based on the principle of the right to self-determination are:

1. the nurse's assistance to individuals in exercising their right to self-determination, through decisions that express the full and unique complexity of their values, and

2. a mode of involvement with patients that necessarily engages the entire self of the nurse. (p. 97)

The complexity of values includes those of the whole family and they must be involved in decision making. When any role holder in the family is dying, the whole family is changed. Yet all the values must be respected, discussed, and shared before satisfying decisions that are right for the whole group are achieved.

This kind of involvement with the family requires the same kinds of characteristics of the nurse as were discussed previously: knowledge of family theory, communication skills, presence, genuineness, and caring. These characteristics help the nurse to assess, plan, and implement the kinds of care that help the family members to make their own decisions, to act on those decisions, and to remain committed to each other.

Commitment to decisions is necessary if the family is to support them. Sometimes, choices that the patient makes can cause the family sorrow, anger, and guilt unless they understand why the decision was made and share in it. For example, if the patient has left final plans that include cremation of the body, and some family members have religious beliefs that prohibit this, conflict will result. Understanding that this is the patient's last wish, and carrying it out as an act of love in spite of one's personal objections, can be healing rather than something to fight about with the siblings.

The nurse does not get into the position of rescuing the patient, making decisions for the patient or family when they are capable of making them (Donahue, 1985). In Mrs. Peterson's case, the nurse does not become the messenger between Mrs. Peterson and her family. She may suggest that family visit more often, but Mrs. Peterson will decide if she really wants that, and it would be appropriate for Mrs. Peterson to ask the family to do so. If the nurse does that, she may find that she gets one message from the family, and a different one from Mrs. Peterson. She may become caught in the middle of a struggle of two groups trying desperately to meet goals of which the other is unaware. It may be helpful to take on the role of facilitator, helping the family and patient to talk with each other. She may role play with Mrs. Peterson, giving her some words to use or ways to ask the family to come in more often. The nurse may be available to the family to answer questions and help them deal with their feelings, but ultimately she must respect their right not to do so if that is what they decide.

Mrs. Peterson needs to be free to make decisions about her own care and relationships without pressure, even if they are in conflict with those of her family. At some point, it is her decision whether to go to a hospital or stay at home with a willing caregiver; about when to stop treatment; and about what she needs to do to maintain the best kind of life for herself for as long as she can. She actively defines the relationship she has with her family. The nurse actively supports these decisions.

Active support for decisions occasionally requires skills in confrontation and negotiation with people or groups outside the family. When hospital or organizational policy prohibits patient choice, the policy is examined for need and relevancy. If it does not serve the safety and patient care needs of others, it may be reviewed to see if it can safely be abrogated. Rigid visiting policies are examples of rules that should be suspended in the interests of patients' rights.

More often than policy problems, intervention is needed because values conflict. The health care system continues to try to preserve life even when the patient may be willing to let go. The nurse who serves as patient advocate must have personal values clearly in mind, and support the patient's right of self-determination. That is not the same thing as agreeing with the decision. Advocacy does not mean that one agrees with the decision made, only with the patient's right to make it. That extends to all of the decisions the patient makes, so long as they do not violate the rights of others or the laws of society. Some nurses are willing to work in the policy or political arenas to bring about social change as a method of patient advocacy.

LEGAL ASPECTS

Advocacy for the patient includes supporting the individual and family in self-determination of treatment choices. There are many reasons why people may not choose the kind of care they want at the end of life. Sometimes they cannot decide because they do not have all the information, or, as discussed previously, they have not discussed the choices fully with family, and believe that the preferred choice will hurt family members in some way. Some people do not realize that there are choices to be made. They may be in denial, or go along with each treatment option as it is presented, believing that the health care team knows the right thing to do at each step in the course of the care. Toward the end of a long period of illness, a patient may become very tired and turn inward. He may find discussion or visits with even the most beloved of family to be an intrusion. In those cases, if treatment options have not been discussed previously, they may be left to a trusted colleague or relative. Internal factors limiting the exercise of the right to self-determination of treatment options include:

- inadequate information
- belief that preferred treatment options will hurt family members because of conflicting beliefs
- denial or other emotional factors
- faith that the health care team knows best
- fatigue
- focus on inner issues rather than care

There are also factors external to the dying person that conspire against self-determination of treatment options. When a person is in an environment or among caregivers who believe that the goal is to avoid death at all costs, it is difficult to call a halt to more tests, more drugs, more assessments. If the physician, the nurse, or family members believe that everything possible should be done to prolong life, it is hard when the patient is sick, tired, and in pain, to say, "No—I have had enough. I want to focus on comfort, saying good-bye, and peace. It's my time, and I am ready."

Organizations have policies that also affect one's right to make decisions about the end of life. Often based in financial considerations and the laws and regulations of the state and federal government, institutions try to protect themselves from litigation or losing large amounts of money in the care of the dying patient. In one state, a hospital refused to allow the removal of a feeding tube for a patient who was dying even though she had requested that it be removed. The hospital based the decision on potential harm to the patient. They may have feared litigation by family members after the death, or being cited by accrediting bodies for unsafe practice. In this case, transfer of the patient to another state with less restrictive laws allowed the patient to choose the preferred care. In other cases, transfer may be unrealistic because of the patient's condition or costs involved. Referral to the hospital ethics committee allows a full hearing of the issues involved. Full hearing may lead to a legally defensible resolution of the issue in the patient's best interest.

Another case involved refusal of the patient's family to be responsible for the continued costs of mechanical ventilation as the precipitating factor in getting the hospital administration to allow the ventilator to be turned off according to the patient's wishes. On occasion, a patient who is receiving some kinds of treatment and is insured privately represents a financial gain to the institution, as when a privately insured patient who is stable but dying a prolonged death is on life-support systems. Factors external to the dying person and family that interfere with the patient's ability to decide the course of treatment include:

- environment in which the goals are always to avoid death at any cost

- personal beliefs of health care professionals or family members that are different from the patient's beliefs

- institutional policies

- state laws and regulations

- reimbursement rates and methods of payment

Advanced Directives

The Patient Self-Determination Act, which went into effect in 1991, requires that all persons who receive funds from Medicare or Medicaid for the care of patients must inform those patients on admission to their services about the right to accept or refuse treatment, and the right to make advanced directives. Advanced directives are legal documents that list those things the patient does not want done in the event he can no longer make decisions for himself (a living will), or gives the right to make decisions about health care to one or more individuals under the same conditions (durable power of attorney for health care). Most organizations offering health care services to the dying now offer standard forms for advanced directives if the patient does not have one already made at the time of admission. These are offered to all people, not only those with Medicare reimbursement.

Standard forms for living wills do not always list everything a patient might wish to include. It is acceptable and in some situations to be encouraged that a person write on the form in handwriting the additional things requested. It is important to recognize that the person has the right to use this format to request treatment, not just to limit it. For example, a patient may request that care specifically include hydration and nutrition by any means, pain relief, and treatment aimed at maximal comfort. Another example is a patient who may wish to be resuscitated up to three times (if possible) before abandoning those kinds of efforts. Patients do not have the right to demand treatment from those unable or unwilling to provide care they believe is medically futile. For example, if a cardiac arrest occurs and is unwitnessed, and the patient is found dead sometime later, starting CPR would be foolish even if the patient had wished it.

The living will is also used to limit treatment. A list of treatments often limited by those who are dying includes:

- mechanical ventilation
- cardiopulmonary resuscitation
- invasive diagnostic tests
- antibiotics for infections
- surgical procedures (include or exclude those used for pain control, such as sympathectomy)

- tube feeding

- dialysis

- intravenous infusion

- blood

Some people prefer not to list options about the specific treatments to be allowed or disallowed if they are unable to make decisions for themselves. They prefer to make decisions on a day-to-day basis for as long as possible, and then ask someone they trust to continue making the decisions as they see fit. A durable power of attorney for health care is a legal document giving the right to make those decisions to a named person or a prioritized list of people (e.g., spouse, eldest child, youngest child, aunt, in that order). Asking a person to make those kinds of life-and-death decisions is a huge act of trust, and confers a great responsibility on the person named. The person taking the responsibility should be fully informed of the patient's beliefs about treatment at the end of life, and feel comfortable that she knows what the patient would want. The need for clear communication between the two, and belief systems that allow the patient's choices to be fulfilled without violating the decision maker's conscience, is obvious.

A living will may be changed at any time. A nurse who is present when a patient expresses a wish to change the components of a living will has an obligation to report that and to provide the means to do so in writing. Oral statements are legally binding in most states, but should be heard by more than one person. The organization generally has someone familiar with advanced directives who can provide new forms or help a patient alter the old ones. Hospital chaplains often perform this role.

Prudent people make advanced directives long before the need arrives, even before any diagnosis of illness. People who are dying often believe they know how much time they have and procrastinate about writing the advanced directive. Even those with terminal diagnoses have no guarantee about life tomorrow. A person living at home with a terminal disease can be treated in a trauma center for injuries received in an automobile accident sustained on the way to the doctor's office. The trauma team will not know that the advanced directive exists unless there is a wallet card indicating where the directive is, who to call about it, or other information about it. To have a choice, the nature of the choice must be shared. Advanced directives of either type do no good if no one knows the document has been made.

When writing the document (or filling in the form) at least two witnesses who are not beneficiaries of the person's estate should sign the directive. Sometimes the nurse is asked to be a witness. Copies should be given to a trusted family member, a doctor or a lawyer, and others told who has the copy in case of need. The document needs to be reviewed and updated on a regular basis to be sure it still reflects what the signer wants to happen. If a family member or friend believes that a person who wrote an advanced directive many years ago has changed desires, and has some testimony by others to that effect, that friend may have the court suspend the directive. Advanced directives should be initialed and dated after review each year to document the current wishes of the person making the directive.

Health care professionals are required to abide by the advanced care directive unless the patient is told beforehand that one or more of the provisions are against the policy of the institution or group. In that case, they must inform the patient in writing, and in case of conflict, follow state law. Sometimes institutions or state offices (e.g., the Governor's office) have ombudsmen who can arbitrate such conflicts. The ombudsman will see that all legal rights are protected. Other people who can help resolve conflict include the hospital administrator, risk management officer, hospital chaplain or other clergy, and the hospital ethics committee. The ethics committee is composed of a variety of people from several disciplines, including nursing, medicine, theology or philosophy, the community, and sometimes other interested people. They review ethical issues on a case-by-case basis, acting for society in determining all ethical options and facilitating decision making, balancing the needs and rights of all parties.

For the dying person, it is wise to know hospital or hospice or institutional policy as it relates to the advanced directive before being admitted. For example, hospice often does not provide cardiopulmonary resuscitation (CPR) for those who die while hospice personnel are present. That fact is shared with patients before admission to hospice. If a living will specifies that CPR is wanted, hospice may not be the best choice of care facility. Or a patient may want to have someone in addition to hospice personnel be present during acute episodes to provide CPR. The patient may decide to enter the hospital when death is near, so that CPR will be done. Health care institutions/organizations must record the fact that a patient has made an advanced directive. That record is found on patients' charts.

The widely reported cases of Karen Ann Quinlan and Nancy Cruzan showed the enormous effort it can take families to get the legal system to allow them to discontinue certain life-support measures. In both cases, the young women were diagnosed to be in a persistent vegetative state, or irreversible coma, and needed supportive care to survive. Neither of the young women had made a living will, but families of both women believed that they knew their wishes regarding living the way they were living. The family of Nancy Cruzan wanted to stop the artificial hydration and feeding that was keeping her alive. The family of Karen Ann Quinlan wanted to stop the respirator ventilating her. After Karen Ann Quinlan's ventilator was removed, she lived another nine years. The families were mired in the legal system for years, at tremendous burden, before reaching a satisfactory conclusion. People who know they are dying can spare their families this burden.

The legal principles defined in part because of these two cases include:

- There is a constitutional right of competent adult patients to be free of unwanted medical treatment.

- This right continues even if the patient is subsequently unable to make medical decisions.

- Different states may have different standards to determine if the patients left information that would clearly show their desire to be treated or not to be treated in different circumstances.

- The state has an interest in preserving life.

- The United States Supreme Court recognized the enforceability of advanced directives. (Hill & Shirley, 1992, pp. 5–11)

Not having an advanced directive means not having a choice. End-of-life wishes may not be honored, even if they are known, if they are not recorded. If family or others know what the wishes are, they must find ways to prove them by testimony of people who heard the patient say what was wanted, or find diaries or other written records expressing choice. This requires more time, money, energy, and emotion by loved ones.

SUMMARY

As simple as it sounds, telling the truth, standing up for your patients and their families, and knowing how they can protect their rights are very simple, yet profound values upon which to build a healing relationship. Truth and advocacy are both rooted in the need to have adequate and accurate information in order to make decisions, and the right to self-determination is more important than the paternalistic pattern of protecting patients from painful knowledge. That kind of paternalism leads to anxiety, lack of trust, and hopelessness, with people often imagining things to be much worse than they really are. Society has encoded the right to self-determination into law, providing several means by which people can express their preferences in end-of-life issues. These rights should be exercised with consultation with the family.

References

Donahue, P. (1985). Advocacy. In G. Bulechek & J. McCloskey (Eds.), *Nursing interventions: Treatments for nursing diagnoses.* Philadelphia: W. B. Saunders Co.

Gadow, S. (1980). An ethical model for assisting patients with treatment decisions. In C. B. Wong & J. Swazey (Eds.), *Dilemmas of dying.* Boston: G. K. Hall Medical Publishers, Inc.

Hill, T. P., & Shirley, D. (1992). *A good death: Taking more control at the end of your life.* Reading, MA: Addison Wesley.

Kübler-Ross, E. (1969). *On death and dying.* New York: McMillan.

Livingston, D. & Williamson, C. (1985). Truth Telling. In G. Bulechek & J. McCloskey (Eds.), *Nursing interventions: Treatments for nursing diagnoses.* Philadelphia: W. B. Saunders Co.

RESOURCES FOR
THE DYING AND
THEIR FAMILIES

9

THE NEED

Many organizations help people who are dying. Some of their goals are to help dying people

- achieve goals at the end of life,
- care for themselves or family members at home,
- grieve after the death of a loved one, or
- find alternative treatments that compliment medical care and help the dying person remain comfortable and at peace.

This chapter focuses on a few large, national resource groups. Three of these groups are part of the federal government and include the Veteran's Administration System, the National Institutes of Health, and Medicare. Hospice is discussed, and a few other large organizations that commonly provide help to dying people are mentioned. A nurse with a strong professional network and local involvement in a health care community can be creative in using these resources to help a dying person live well until death.

Arthur's Helpers

Arthur, a gay man with Acquired Immune Deficiency Syndrome (AIDS), was having a hard time. His health care was provided by a free clinic, but surgery was required and the local hospital did not want to admit him for the procedure. Surgeons were not willing to operate because they feared the virus. When he did find a county hospital willing to do the surgery, he was very sick, and a prolonged convalescence of at least six weeks was expected. He was discharged in ten days, unable to care for himself. His prognosis was guarded. He would recover from the surgery, but no one could predict the course of the AIDS.

A coalition of gay men and lesbian women had organized a self-help group to help people like Arthur. They sent members of the group to clean his house and leave two meals a day, keep the lawn mowed, and do the shopping, as long as Arthur needed that help. He also had a driver to take him to his follow-up appointments. He recovered, was able to care for himself in about three weeks (except for yard work, which required two months further help), and was relatively well for another year. Provision of simple housekeeping services and food were all that he required.

FINDING RESOURCES

Many people who have a terminal illness need help. Some, like Arthur, live alone but are members of a group who have the resources to assist their members. Others have families or live with people who need basic information on how to help with both physical care and provision of basic human needs. Some families are unable to provide such help because they are worn out, or are themselves ill. Other families are dysfunctional, barely able to care for members of the family when they are healthy. The impending death immobilizes and paralyzes the family, as discussed previously. The nurse's role in healing the dying becomes one of forging or supporting connections and relationships between the dying patient and groups or individuals willing to help.

Connecting the patient with the resources needed for care requires knowledge of resources and the ability to either recommend them to patients who will use them independently or to make the referrals. A list of useful national resources, both hot lines and addresses of national organizations that have information, publications, referral resources, or specific kinds of assistance available to individuals, can be found in appendix 3. Local organizations vary significantly in the type and amount of assistance that can be offered to individuals.

Nurses can get listings of helpful local groups in several ways. National organizations will refer inquirers to local affiliates. Local libraries often maintain lists (sometimes for sale) of community organizations. These lists are updated annually or biannually, usually include phone numbers, and may be categorized into a section on health for easy reference. The League of Women Voters and local chapters of national organizations like the American Red Cross sometimes have lists of agencies that they use for public relations or information. They may charge a small fee for access to the lists.

Nurses who work for large institutions or organizations generally have access to people who know about the resources in the geographic area. Case managers, discharge planners, social workers, and even volunteers often know about agencies or groups who provide care, information, or support to dying people. They keep resource lists with current telephone numbers, criteria for enrollment of patients, and costs. They can contact a long list of care providers, including home health agencies, hospice services, home nutrition services, and agencies that provide special services like respiratory care, parenteral nutrition, physical therapy, occupational therapy, homemakers, personal care attendants, financial aid, and respite care. Barriers to using these services include availability, cost, and accurate assessment of need.

One useful way of identifying resources is to remain a part of an organization or network of local nurses who know the resources available and will share that information. Members of specialty organizations often find that one of the most useful benefits of membership is sharing the knowledge of resources others in the group have found. Those resources may include organizations, representatives of companies that give away sample products for testing, alternative care providers, or people with special information who are willing to give educational programs. One nurse who practiced Therapeutic Touch (TT) in a southeastern state was cited in a national publication. She received a call from a Canadian man concerned about his wife who had been recently diagnosed with breast cancer. He wanted to know how to find a person who practiced TT in Manitoba, and how to go about evaluating alternative health care in general. Because the nurse was a member of the Professional Nurse Healers and had received a directory of practitioners, she was able to refer him to members living close to his hometown who could help him. Directories of nurses and other health care personnel with specialized practices (e.g., diabetes nurse educators) can be very useful.

Patients, too, often find resources that they are entitled to use. Companies they work for may provide benefits. Lodges or groups like the Shriners provide care to children if certain qualifications are met. Religious affiliation may provide access to resources. One church raised $50,000 to help a member get on a heart transplant list, another provided visitors to a man who was dying and needed to talk. Parish nursing is developing in some areas as a means of churches addressing more comprehensive care needs of parishioners. These nurses may be able to find sitters, volunteer drivers, and other helpers for the family or patient who needs help.

MAKING REFERRALS

Referral to an agency that provides direct care on a fee-for-service basis is probably the easiest and most common approach to provision of care for the dying for those who can afford it or who have insurance that covers it. Gaps in referrals and lack of continuity of care between hospital and home can occur for several reasons, with lack of monetary resources comprising only part of the problem.

Persons treated in a large referral hospital may live in a different geographical area, and the staff of the hospital may not know community resources available there. These hospitals generally refer to a primary care service. That service may not be aware of all the needs of the dying individual related to treatments rendered at the referral center. For that reason, careful documentation is a crucial part of the referral process, with a telephone call between discharge nurse and new agency a very helpful way to clarify what treatments were given, how care is being done, and what the nurse believes will be needed at the home or place of discharge. If a visit by the home care provider to the patient before the discharge from the hospital is possible, it is very useful for planning purposes and for getting any physician's orders needed for medications and treatments. The referral process requires that the discharge nurse has done a careful assessment of the patient and family, both needs and strengths, and has thoughtfully planned for future needs. Networks of providers, including nurses, are continually being created both formally and informally, and they aid the referral process.

Unfortunately, too often the need for services is not apparent while a person is hospitalized or receiving active treatment. Even if the need is assessed appropriately, once the person is discharged and the needs change, a reassessment may not be done. For example, a primary care practitioner following a patient through office visits may not be told of nonmedical problems, like caregiver fatigue or diminishing functional ability with regard to food preparation, and may not ask about it. So people with serious needs are in the community and do not know where to go for help. Help can be classified as either information services or agencies/people who provide care.

GOVERNMENT

Organizations may be grouped by type of ownership: profit-making, government, or not-for-profit organizations. Profit-making services are often included as home health services within a corporation devoted to health care. They can be found in each community, and often reflect the social and economic background of that community. An example is the fact that health food stores may be found in communities with socially sophisticated, upwardly mobile young professionals, while no such options are in evidence in inner city neighborhoods.

Resources for care of dying people are provided by both the United States government and various state and local governments. Two of the largest U.S. government programs that provide direct services to people are the V.A./military system and the Department of Health and Human Services (HHS). HHS is responsible for the Health Care Financing Agency (HCFA), administrators of the Medicare program, the Social Security Administration, which manages payments for disabled people as well as aged or blind people, and the U.S. Public Health Service, which is responsible for the Agency for Health Care Policy and Research.

Veteran's Administration

The federal government has programs useful for military and retired military personnel who are dying, whether or not the reason for the final illness is service-connected. Often found within Veteran's Administration Hospitals, services for the dying include both inpatient and outpatient medical care, prescribed drugs and equipment like ostomy supplies, treatments, and financial services. Offices within the Veteran's Administration (V.A.) will help veterans find out if they are eligible for care within the V.A. system. Programs of care vary between hospitals, some providing inpatient hospice-like care, others being only acute care facilities. Most will provide needed medication. Veterans' groups often volunteer time and resources for their military compatriots, visiting them and bringing toiletries, entertainment, and a sense of belonging to the larger group. In the natural reminiscence that takes place, people resolve many old issues.

Mr. Bower's Buddies

It was a day Mr. Bower usually tried to forget. Years before, in Korea, his platoon had been fired on, and several of his friends had been wounded. Two of them had died. During the fight, Mr. Bower had distinguished himself (he never said what he did), and was commended for his heroism. On the anniversary of the fight, three of the men who had been there and now lived in Mr. Bower's city showed up at the V.A. hospital and had a ceremony to honor those who had fought. Remembering the two who had died, and being honored for helping the living, Mr. Bower finally came to a peace about that incident in his life. His comrades in arms, through their thoughtfulness to the whole group, helped one dying member to find peace.

Research Information from the Federal Government

The National Institutes of Health (NIH) are supported by the U.S. government for the purpose of research and have a variety of treatment programs underway at all times. Doctors working in the National Cancer Institute (NCI), National Institute of Mental Health (NIMH), Heart Lung and Blood, and others admit patients to rigidly controlled studies. They find patients to admit to their research programs through other practicing physicians. People wishing to fight their disease by becoming study subjects should ask their physicians for information, or ask the doctor to call the National Institute of Health that relates to their problem to determine if any of the current studies are appropriate for them. The National Cancer Institute maintains a database called Physicians Data Query, or PDQ, which lists protocols and study information on at least 85 treatments, with 1,000 protocols and 12,000 physicians (Lesko, 1994).

The U.S. government maintains many information services related to health care. An example is the Agency for Health Care Policy and Research, which publishes guidelines for treatment on such topics as pain control, pressure sores, incontinence, depression, and other problems that commonly complicate the care of dying people. Information for patients or clinicians can be obtained without cost (see table 9.1).

Agency for Health Care Policy and Research

Clinical guidelines relevant to the care of the dying are available from this agency by writing to:

AHCPR Clearinghouse
P.O. Box 8547
Silver Springs, MD 20907

or calling 1-800-358-9295. Guidelines available include:

Pressure Ulcers in Adults: Prediction and Prevention
Urinary Incontinence in Adults
Evaluation and Management of Early HIV Infection
Acute Pain Management: Operative or Medical Procedures and Trauma
Management of Cancer Pain: Adults

Social Security Administration

Information about financial assistance available through this agency can be obtained by writing to:

Department of Health and Human Services
Social Security Administration
Baltimore, MD 21235

Booklets available include:

Understanding Social Security
Medicare
Disability
A Guide to SSI for Groups and Organizations
Survivors

All of these resources are available without charge.

TABLE 9.1   *Selected Print Resources, Government*

Hot lines are maintained to provide access to information, offer referral services, and sometimes provide financial assistance. Private agencies as well as the government maintain hot lines as efficient methods of distributing health care information. The National Health Information Center (P.O. Box 1133, Washington, D.C., 20013) can send a publication catalog. Two of the publications listed are a list of selected Federal Health Information Clearinghouses and Information Centers and Toll-free Numbers for Health Information. Appendix 3 lists a few of those that relate to common problems of the dying patient or to certain disease states. Each nurse will want to check the current telephone number of the relevant hot lines in a current directory of 800 numbers or through directory assistance, and keep the information updated in a resource file specific to the case load.

Local Government

State and local governments vary by locale in terms of provision of care and information that help dying patients. A variety of social programs help to feed and care for people who lack the financial means to help themselves, though programs are limited and never enough to meet all the needs. Food banks, food stamps, Medicaid funds, county hospitals for indigent patients (often supported in part by both state and county), community health clinics (including those for specific diagnoses like AIDS), transportation vouchers for trips to the hospital, and home health aid programs are found in many localities. Each governmental unit has its own set of regulations and requirements for enrollment. Quasi-governmental agencies, those supported in part by the government through grants and other means, like senior citizen centers in some places, may have volunteers and other programs that support dying people, with different requirements for enrollment.

States provide regulation and monitoring of care facilities and care providers for the protection of the public. There is a mechanism in each state that receives and investigates complaints about substandard care given to patients, should a family be concerned about that kind of event. The State Board of Nursing for the state serves that function for complaints about nurses. A national Disciplinary Data Base (DDB) is maintained listing practitioners (including physicians and nurses) who have been disciplined in their states or who have malpractice claims filed against them. Facilities and agencies should be licensed and regularly monitored for adherence to standards.

NONGOVERNMENTAL ORGANIZATIONS

Voluntary agencies provide support to people who meet their criteria. Since each agency has different criteria that change frequently, the search for support can be confusing and frustrating. That is why consulting with people who do discharge planning or home health is often a useful first step—they have up-to-date information and can save many phone calls and letters. The best-known and most comprehensive set of services offered specifically for dying patients is offered by Hospice, a fee-for-service, nonprofit organization.

Hospice

Hospice is not a place, it is a "well-coordinated set of services intended to relieve or ease the varied symptoms or side effects of a terminal illness" (Beresford, 1993). Hospice staff and volunteers help people live well until they die. The overall goal is to provide comfort and care for people who are dying and their families. It usually occurs in the home, but some inpatient hospice units exist.

St. Christopher's in Sydenham, England is usually considered the first modern hospice. Hospice care first developed when human beings formed settled communities and began to care for sick people. Many had religious orientations, such as those associated with Egyptian, Oriental, Greek, and Roman temples that were used as refuges for travelers and the sick. Christianity and Islam both supported the care of the sick as a religious duty, and built peaceful hospice structures throughout their respective territories. Crusaders spread the hospice idea by helping to build hospices on their way to and from crusades, and by using them when weary and attempting to return home to England (Siebold, 1992, p.16). The hospices provided respite and kindness, but not medical care.

During the Dark Ages, many hospices disappeared and others became almshouses, places where disease was not controlled and no one went if they had a choice. When modern medicine developed, hospices became hospitals, devoted to the cure of disease. But a few hospices dedicated to the care of the incurably ill continued or were reborn. In 1879, Our Lady's Hospice opened to provide palliative care for the terminally ill, the first facility created under religious auspices to do so in the nineteenth century. Sister Mary Aikenhead, an Irish nun who had worked with Florence Nightingale and was knowledgeable about the French hospices associated with the order of St. Vincent De Paul, was credited with being the inspiration for the opening of that hospice (Siebold, 1992).

Two women became charismatic and outspoken advocates of the hospice movement in the 1950s and 1960s. Dr. Cicely

Saunders developed a comprehensive program of physical, emotional, and spiritual care for palliation of symptoms and support of people who were dying and their families. Dr. Elizabeth Kübler-Ross supported such a movement based on her studies of the process of dying, the identified need for such support, and the obvious benefits to those people and their families when such support was given. Through the efforts of Dr. Saunders, St. Christopher's Hospice in England became a model of care for the dying, a place to demonstrate how to care for people who could not be cured. Through the efforts of Dr. Kübler-Ross, the awareness of the emotional and spiritual needs of terminally ill people was popularized.

Americans and the English have different sets of values related to dying, so it is not possible to simply move the English system of hospice to the United States. At St. Christopher's, no vital signs are taken, no I.V.s are given, and few blood tests are done. For Americans, this appears to be neglect. Americans are not accepting of lack of access to technology and are not generally accepting of death. In addition, Saunders writes of differences between American and British physicians, stating that as a British physician, she was willing to carry out, not write, orders for ancillary staff (Siebold, 1992, p. 71). Hers is an interdisciplinary approach, and the doctor is not always the team leader.

The American hospice movement, then, developed differently from the British system. There is not one hospice, but each has developed locally according to the goals, values, and resources of the community it serves. A National Hospice Organization serves as a clearinghouse of information, and can refer people to local hospice services. Following is a set of objectives with which most hospices in the United States agree:

- The patient participates in the treatment and maintains independence and control as long as possible.

- The patient and family are a unit of care. When the patient dies, the family may need continued care for a period of time.

- The care team is interdisciplinary.

- Pain management and symptom control are major goals.

- Care is affordable.

Enrollment in a hospice generally requires that a patient's values are similar to the hospice. That means that the patient is seeking comfort-oriented care rather than aggressive treatment aimed at extending life at all costs. Some hospice teams refuse to give cardiopulmonary resuscitation should death occur when they are present, and the patient must understand that this service is not provided. In the past, some hospices required the patient to sign DNR (do not resuscitate) orders prior to enrollment, but new laws about living wills and other end-of-life issues (the Patient Self-Determination Act of 1991) make that a questionable legal issue. Some people feel it is not legal or ethical to require a patient to surrender rights (in this case, the right to CPR) in order to receive the kind of care otherwise desired. Enrollment into hospice is fully explained and patient, family, and patient's physician all consent in writing to hospice care.

Other criteria for enrollment into hospice are:

- Medical diagnosis of a terminal disease, with a prognosis of six months to a year (Medicare requirements are more specific, and change from time to time).

- There must be a caregiver present, usually a family member or significant person in the patient's life, though sometimes a church or organization may take responsibility for caring for a member.

- Hospice care must be provided in a safe setting: safe for patient, family, and hospice worker.

The interdisciplinary team members of a hospice unit assigned to one patient depend on the needs of the individual. Teams meet regularly to develop, maintain, review, and carry out a plan of care and treatment for the patient. The team works together to achieve consensus on the plan of care so that each team member is committed to the same goals. They organize themselves to visit the patient on different days so that the patient is seen as often as possible. They are careful to document all care for communication as well as for legal reasons.

A typical early arrangement might be for the nurse-case manager to see the patient for evaluation initially and once a week; a care attendant to provide personal care three times a week; and a physical therapist to teach the family safe ways of exercising the patient on an alternate day. The patient or family can call these team members any time, usually asking the nurse to coordinate the calls. The patient's physician, fully a member of the team, follows the patient through office visits and by phone with the registered nurse when the patient's condition changes and new orders are needed.

Volunteers are also members of the team, even when they spend most of their time in the hospice office. When they are assigned to a family, they may be used to sit with the patient and give caregivers a few hours off, or they may provide transportation to the doctor's office or other treatment center. They may also walk the dog, deliver medicines, or baby-sit. Most often, they make the family situation easier to manage.

An integral part of the team, the social worker focuses on the financial environment and relationships. Some functions overlap those of the nurse, and if the social worker and the nurse work well together, the overlapping competencies can be a strength of the team. For example, sometimes both the nurse and the social worker are qualified to do supportive counseling. The

---

Help families get financial services to which they are entitled; for example:

• Medicare

• Medicaid

• Social Security

• Food stamps

• Insurance payments

• Company benefits

Help families with legal issues, such as:

• How to get a will made

• Information on advanced directives, living wills

• Informed consent

Referrals for community services, such as:

• Funeral homes

• Local branches of organizations that can provide equipment like wheelchairs or hospital beds, flags for coffins, and other anticipated needs

Family conferences to resolve conflict, and other types of supportive counseling in collaboration with other team members who are able to offer counseling services.

TABLE 9.2 *Hospice Social Worker Responsibilities*

hospice chaplain may also be qualified to do counseling. In this case, the team will decide who takes on the responsibility for this task based on the relationship with the family and other responsibilities. Other responsibilities of the social worker are listed in table 9.2, and of the registered nurse in table 9.3.

Bereavement services are a part of hospice. People who have worked together to ease the death of another, families and hospice team together, have gone through a shared, intense emotional experience together. Counseling is often available, and meetings at annual candlelight remembrances or other planned events are helpful to both groups of people—just to see how they are doing. Children, in particular, are cared for in groups or sometimes summer camps, so that they can meet and discuss loss of a loved one with other children in a nurturing environment.

Coordinates care
- Skilled assessment of patient and family
- Communication with physician
- Communication with other team members
- Follows up with documentation
- Calls team meetings, generally leads them

Provides direct patient care
- Pain control
- Psychological support
- Skilled nursing care requirements
- On-call coverage for crises and to be with patient and family at the time of patient's death
- Family grief counseling after the patient's death

Education
- Patient
- Family
- Care team

TABLE 9.3   *Registered Nurse Responsibilities*

Other Organizations

The American Cancer Society maintains a room across the street from a large medical facility for adult cancer patients who come from out of town for cancer treatments. Nearby, the Ronald McDonald House may be used by children and their families for the same purpose. It is supported by private and corporate funds in many cities. A funeral home offers the services of a Master's degreed bereavement counselor for a month following the death of a loved one as a natural part of the care they give to customers. The counselor provides group sessions to help family members talk about their loss and move through the immediate period of bereavement. These are examples of private and corporate recognition and funding of resources useful to dying people in one American city.

Hospice services have a clear and coherent set of purposes and guidelines, though local groups vary in some procedural and funding issues. Other organizations are formed around other parameters of care, most often a disease (like cancer), a system (like the heart or kidney or liver), a procedure (like transplantation), or a symptom (like pain). National organizations exist to address many of these problems. If a patient who is dying has needs that are unfulfilled and the family seems unable to meet them, community outreach from these groups is often a viable alternative. Communities exist to care for their members. Creative nurses look for resources for patients from them, if not directly, then through social service workers or volunteers in the agency where the nurse works. As with the funeral director who initiated bereavement counseling for customers, other entrepreneurs in the community are becoming health conscious and willing to offer increasing levels of services to customers. These businesspeople need only to be asked by consumers of their services or products for help that they can give.

SUMMARY

Meeting the needs of dying patients and their families is a part of healing the dying. A caring professional expertly brings to their care the things people need to be able to maintain their quality of life and achieve a sense of peace and continuity of life through family and community. The resources needed vary greatly, taking the form of financial and physical resources like food, equipment, and money, together with people who have knowledge and ability to help with grief and bereavement in all its forms.

The United States government provides major resources in the form of veterans' care, Medicare for aged and disabled citizens, and research plans and care for those who qualify. Large national organizations provide information and more limited access to care, equipment, and services. Hospice services are available in most areas for people who are dying and wish to focus on palliative care. Appendix 3 lists hot lines and resource clearinghouses that may be useful to those seeking resources. Networking with health care professionals who have knowledge of resources in a community is the most effective way to learn of resources.

References

Beresford, L. (1993). *The hospice handbook: A complete guide.* Boston: Little, Brown & Co.

Lesko, M. (1994). *Lesko's info-power* (2nd ed.). Detroit, MI: Visible Ink Press.

Siebold, C. (1992). *The hospice movement: Easing death's pains.* New York: Twayne Publishers.

4 | SPECIAL CASES

10 | WHEN SPECIAL PEOPLE DIE

FAMILY

Nurses care for people who, in their dying, present special problems or have special needs. Some of those problems may belong to the nurse when the patient is someone close, like a parent, spouse, child, or friend. Sometimes those patients have a stigmatizing illness, like Sudden Infant Death Syndrome (SIDS) or Acquired Immune Deficiency Syndrome (AIDS). Sometimes the patients are victims of violence, like homicide or suicide, and the nurse is concerned with perceived injustice in the world. Sometimes the death is that of a colleague. When death occurs to these people, there are often special considerations in their care and in care for the caregivers.

Death of Parents of Adult Children

The death of a parent is often difficult and complicated because of the history of relationship, and the fact that the loss extends beyond the loss of an individual. For some people, the relationship with the parent is the most stable relationship in life, the place where they can always turn for unconditional love. For others, the relationship has been confusing.

While it is generally accepted that in the natural order of events parents die before their children, there is always a sense of loss that transcends the death of one person. There is the loss of opportunity to respond, to tell the parent of one's love, and to thank the parent for the many small things given or shared. There is the loss of the opportunity to share significant secrets of life. One man regretted that he had never shared the fact that he was gay with his father, and would never know how his father would have reacted to that fact. He continually built fantasies about how he thought his father would have felt, sometimes thinking that the father would have been supportive and loving, other times believing the father would have rejected him. There was no way to confirm either scenario after the death of the father. Somehow the relationship was never complete because the secrets were never shared (Akner, 1993).

For one daughter, the death of a mother meant she lost contact with relatives in Sweden, because she had never learned the language. The loss of family ties in the old country was significant to her. Some adult children believe they have never measured up to a parent's standards, and now will never be able to prove themselves. Or they feel guilty for things left undone. For children who have no siblings and are unmarried, the death of a parent may be the death of the whole family. Even adult children may feel abandoned, especially if parent and child never talked about death.

Some children have accepted the caregiving role for their parents for years. The death of a parent who has been the focus of a person's attentions for several years may leave that person feeling less needed by others. It also leaves a hole in the daily schedule, and a need to make choices about what to do with time, how to form new relationships, and decisions about a person's responsibility to others. A person's meaning in life may have been bound to her caretaking activities, and without that responsibility, life loses its meaning.

In the time preceding the death of a parent, hard decisions may have been made. Treatment decisions, like discontinuing noxious medications, placing parents in care institutions, withdrawing life-support systems, or using needed family resources for care when cure seems hopeless may all burden the family grieving the loss of a parent. If the parent has left explicit instructions for these decisions, it may be easier for the adult children.

When parents die, there is always a change in family relationships. If the family has been dysfunctional, it may have been one parent who kept the peace. If so, someone else must take on that role if the family is to have peace. Or the relationships will need to be repatterned so there is no need for a peacemaker. That is unlikely to happen without help. A mature, functioning family will grieve together, find ways to grow closer, and realign roles.

There are several things that a nurse can do to help adult children who have lost a parent. The first is to realize that the loss is always significant. There is no such thing as finding solace in words like, "He was 95 years old and led a long and healthy life. This was a good way to go." A child of 70 years of age who had a parent for all of those 70 years will be confronted with mortality and feel alone. There will be a need for a period of grieving and then a connection with others for healing to occur. Silence, allowing tears, giving time for the person to remain with a body if necessary to say good-bye, a caring touch on the shoulder, or holding a person's hand all reflect a caring presence and a genuine desire to share the loss. Sharing last words the child may not have heard or a funny story that the parent shared with the nurse about a family member may be a good connection.

An adult who has lost a parent needs to identify the extent of the losses in his life and how to deal with those losses. Support groups for adults who have lost parents are often effective, usually lasting four to six weeks, and helping people through some of the intense grief and issues of their own mortality. Clergy, counselors who understand bereavement issues, and family members who are coping well may be excellent resources for follow-up. If depression follows prolonged grieving, professional help is recommended. The nurse who maintains an ongoing relationship with the family, perhaps through hospice or other follow-up services of the organization, should be alert for signs of prolonged grieving, depression, or suicide.

Parents who have prepared well, discussed death with the children, and were able to meet the criteria for a "good death," dying alert and without pain, in comfort and having completed the tasks of saying good-bye and accomplishing goals, leave a model of how to die well. If they have prepared financially, left final directives, and shown their children how they fit into the intergenerational family (their place in the interconnectedness of people through the generations), they help the children see death as personally less fearsome, a normal part of life. But they cannot take away the sense of loss and separation. That is a part of love.

Death of Parents of Younger Children

Children who are not adults and lose their parent or parents have a different set of reactions and needs. Not only do they suffer the trauma of separation and loss for a loved one, but there is a "serious developmental interference" (Buckingham, 1990). Their security is threatened. They do not know how to act or what to do when the parent is not there to do the things the child has come to trust that the parent will do. As one small child said when informed of a death, "She never did that before."

Children are unable to grieve intensely for long periods of time, so they have short periods of intense grief and crying, punctuated by periods of watching TV, playing, and doing other things that the adults around them may feel are inappropriate. Yet the periods that appear to be denial are probably protective, giving the child time to think through this new event. Many children regress in their behavior, moving to a previous stage of development. Bed-wetting may recur after a death in a child who had not been wetting the bed for some time. The child may revert to former speech patterns or thumb sucking or other regressive behavior. Like the crying and the TV watching, this is intermittent.

Grieving children often feel guilty, as if they did something to contribute to the death. They need:

- reassurance that they did not cause the death
- the opportunity and encouragement to express their fears and anger
- to be loved and secure
- to accept their own feelings, alien though they may seem

For them, getting on with their lives means continuing to achieve the appropriate developmental tasks for their ages, including a revised understanding of security.

There are two tasks involved in children's grief. Children must release the sad feelings and give up the lost parent (Buckingham, 1990, p. 36). Families are the ideal resource for grieving children, to help with both tasks. However, with the loss of a parent, the whole family is grieving and often finds coping difficult. They can get help from support groups like Hospice, which has a number of programs for grieving children aimed at helping them to express their feelings via drawings, talking with other children, and sending letters to heaven. Nurses are often active in children's support groups, helping children learn to cope with the loss of a parent. Children's hospitals sometimes have children's support groups, which are run by volunteers, nurses, or sometimes social workers.

Grieving children should always be told the truth. Daddy has not just gone away. If he is dead, he is not coming back, and the child should be allowed to grieve that fact. Otherwise, the sense of abandonment and mistrust is hard to overcome, even later in life. If the child has been with a dying patient, seen the body, talked with others about the impending death as the child is able to understand, the grieving will probably be shorter. The child will learn to cope more quickly. The child may have been able to say good-bye. For a child to learn to cope with the death of a loved one, a healing relationship with other family members or caregivers is very important.

Death of a Child

When a child dies, it somehow seems so much worse than when a parent dies. The life seems too short, too unfulfilled. Yet a wise pediatric nurse said to a weeping student nurse who had lost a three-year-old patient, "Every life, no matter how short, is a complete life." This nurse measured life in something other than time.

The dying child has the same needs for healing relationships as any dying person, and needs for comfort, pain control, reassurance, and care. The child may have gone through many remissions, repeated hospitalizations, varied treatment protocols, and periods of feeling well alternating with periods of feeling very unwell. Such a child is able to play with friends and achieve the developmental progress expected some of the time, but not at other times. If the repeated treatment cycles leave the child with less and less energy, a kind of lethargy and perhaps depression are likely. The child is likely to accept the fact of impending death before the parents do, and sometimes feels guilty about that. It is as if the child wants to get it over with, and get on to the next phase of existence (Buckingham, 1990).

Most people who work with dying children know that honesty is the basis of trust, and there is really no question about telling the child that death is probable. The child will know and will ask quite directly if she is going to die, but only if she feels she will get an honest answer and that her question will not hurt the one she asks too much. Asking a parent may not be possible if the child is aware the parent is avoiding the subject and cannot deal with it. The child may ask someone else, like a nurse. When working with a dying child, the nurse should be prepared when the child says something like, "I know I'm going to die." Reflexively denying the possibility is not helpful to the child. Admitting that death is a possibility opens the door to future discussion. The child's questioning should indicate how much and when information should be given. The child may initially be seeking specific information about how much pain is likely or whether a family pet will be present in heaven. Encouraging the child to draw pictures and share the drawings can be helpful. The pictures will often include scenes of the afterlife from the child's point of view. The child can play games about death with dolls to work out feelings, and discuss death with understanding people—other children, teachers, and the family.

If the nurse does discuss death with a child, the family should know that the child is able to discuss the topic. When the family members are able to handle the conversation, they can be helped to share their understanding with the child in conversation. Past experience with death in the family is a building block that can help the family get more direct with each other and with the child about the child's feelings about her own impending death. While it is important to be honest and direct with children to the extent that they seem to want to talk, it is important to realize that as with adults, there is always hope. Neither life nor the time of death is ever certain. The hope may be for a quick end, more time, less pain, or many other things. Children have spiritual needs just as adults do, and often find prayer or meditation a comforting and satisfying thing to do, especially if it has been a routine in the home.

Some older children find meaning in their illness, and a way to fight the illness by discussing it directly with others. Teens share their experiences with peers at camps during the summer or in treatment facilities as they can. Ryan White, a teen dying from AIDS contracted through blood transfusions, was well-known for fighting the injustice of social isolation up to the time of his death. When the school board refused to let him attend school, fearing infection of healthy children, he not only sued the board to allow him to pursue his education, but spoke publicly to lawmakers, other children, and the news media to educate them on the facts of transmission of HIV and how it feels to be dying. He even wrote a book on his experiences (White & Cunningham, 1991). Teens might find it helpful to read his book and know that others have feelings about death that may be quite similar to their own.

Children worry about leaving parents in grief. Some people think that worry can prolong the struggle, preclude a peaceful death. One loving family had a six-year-old son who battled with leukemia for three years. On his last day, he told his mother he didn't want her to be sad, and she would be sad when he died. Later in the day, he began to bleed, and his respirations were agonal. But it seemed he was still struggling for every breath. His mother whispered to him that it might be time for him to let go, and if it was, she wanted him to know that she would always love him, but she and his father would be all right. He immediately stopped struggling, soon slipped into unconsciousness, and peacefully died two hours later. This mother did not hasten the child's death, but she may have made it more comfortable.

Helping parents through the death of a child requires compassion and tolerance. If the death was expected, the family should have decided such issues as organ donation prior to the death. If it was sudden, as in the case of an accident, they will be asked to make important decisions about organ donation, choice of mortuary or funeral home, and other things they may never have thought about with regard to their child. They will be asked to make these decisions during a time of shock. Parents will probably need some time with the child, to be allowed to hold him, and the nurse must be sensitive to their need for support or privacy. They may need family, counselors, or other significant people in their lives, perhaps their own parents. If no one is available, the nurse may call the hospital chaplain or social worker or other person who can help with support and decision making.

Sudden Infant Death Syndrome (SIDS)

SIDS is a special problem because in society, parents are supposed to protect and care for their infants. For most SIDS deaths, defined as the sudden death of an infant who previously appeared healthy, there was no warning of impending death, no way the parents could have known the child needed protection or care. But the parents will experience grief, anger, fear, and guilt. Many parents imagine that others look at them with judgment, wondering how they could have let their child die. The beginning of healing for these parents is the closure of relationship with the infant. After the child has been pronounced dead, the parents need to hold the child, sometimes several times between the death and the funeral. Health care workers are urged to treat the infant's body as a child, keeping it swaddled in a blanket, and holding it like a baby. Leaving it unclothed and unattended on a stretcher or in the back of a mortuary vehicle can be extremely upsetting to parents who continue to be parents and see the infant as needing care and protection (Corr et al., 1991). Parents need to have respectful attention, privacy when requested, and a place to express emotion. Some specific things that can be offered are:

- allowing them to take something of the infant's, like a lock of hair or the baby blanket

- offering to arrange transportation home from the emergency room or to call family members

- keeping them fully informed, including who to call about autopsy results

- making referrals, including the local SIDS network

These parents in particular will be cut off from other parents with young children, and afraid for their other children, existing or planned. They need connection with family and those who understand SIDS. And they need information about subsequent risk of SIDS for other children.

Siblings

The death of a child may have profound effects on siblings. Through the course of a long illness, siblings may have received less attention than the sick child and had strong feelings about perceived lack of love or parental favoritism for the ill child. They may have felt less important than the dying child, even rejected. When that child dies, the sibling often feels guilty, as if negative thoughts or jealously caused the death. The sibling may have lost a good friend, if a close relationship existed with the sick child. The sibling who does not understand the nature of illness may also feel that she will die.

Helping the siblings is much like helping a child understand the death of a parent. They need to be able to express feelings, and ultimately move on in life to achieve their own developmental tasks. Parents should be encouraged and reminded to help these children by talking with them. Appropriate goals are to help them get back into a stable routine, including school or other regular daily activity, and to understand short-term regressive behavior, like fear of the dark, that may be exhibited following the death. Children's support groups, school counselors, and mental health experts are all potential resources for the child who continues to have difficulty.

Death of a Spouse

The death of a spouse, like the death of a parent or the death of a child, is always unique and seems devastating. Two human beings have chosen to create a life together that no one else could have created. When one is left, the life is different, often significantly so. How a surviving spouse copes depends on the nature of the life created together, the nature of the death, and the environment. Factors associated with spouses who do not move through the grief and continue to have difficulty for a prolonged time include:

- sudden untimely death of the spouse
- multiple losses
- high dependency on the deceased
- perceived lack of support
- poor health prior to bereavement (Benoliel, 1991)

A nursing responsibility is to identify these risk factors and to act to lessen the effects. For example, in chapter 3, Mrs. J. lost her husband, and only a few months later chose to have heart surgery. She was coping with her poor health prior to bereavement. Her decision was supported by the nurse.

People who have created a life together in which there is a mutual dependency will each have deficits when living life alone. For example, an aging wife who depended on her husband to drive will have transportation problems to solve. A young husband who does not know how to feed a young child may need to learn to warm a bottle. If one spouse handled all the family finances and dies first, the other will need to learn about money—where it is, how much there is, and how to get it. Referral to social workers may be helpful or family financial planners, if available.

In the time immediately after the death, the communication skill of listening helps to identify the importance of ideas such as, "What will I do now?" It is important to realize that the person may not be asking for direction concerning who to call or what other immediate actions are necessary. The person may be asking, "What do I do with the rest of my life?" Focusing on the immediate problems may be a way to avoid thinking about long-term changes for a while, but it may also be necessary. The skillful nurse knows when to help the grieving spouse move forward. A discussion of helping all people through grief is found in chapter 3. The surviving spouse will redefine the meaning of an individual life, perhaps seek meaning in death, and create a new life without the spouse.

STIGMATIZING ILLNESS

Stigmatization by society is the characterization of some diseases or problems as a disgrace, in some way bad or morally reprehensible. It leads to people who have those problems becoming isolated, lonely, unsupported, and often starts a downward spiral toward decreasing health. A new widow or widower often experiences social isolation because the places they visited with a spouse do not welcome unattached people. Widowhood may become stigmatizing in some settings. Hopefully, after the death of a spouse, a person grieves, recovers, and soon finds a new circle of friends, and the stigma can be overcome. More difficult to handle is the stigmatization of Acquired Immune Deficiency Syndrome (AIDS), violence, or suicide. AIDS, in particular, is the stigmatizing disease of the 1990s, as tuberculosis was earlier in the century.

Acquired Immune Deficiency Syndrome (AIDS)

The stigmatization that comes from having AIDS is due to the fact that the first identified groups of People With AIDS (PWAs) were members of socially unacceptable minority groups (in the United States), or engaged in socially unacceptable behavior: intravenous drug users, gay men, and poor Haitians. Though AIDS strikes heterosexual people, people from any country, and people without high-risk behavior, it continues to be stigmatizing and isolating because it is viewed as incurable and contagious. People are afraid of AIDS.

AIDS is probably not as contagious as once thought. If a person is not engaging in high-risk behavior, even working with AIDS patients on a daily basis poses very little risk, almost none if universal precautions as established by the Centers for Disease Control are always used. High-risk groups include anyone who has sex with another person other than in the context of a monogamous relationship (by both partners), receives unscreened blood products, sticks themselves with contaminated needles, or is infected through skin breaks by contaminated blood or body fluids. There are a few cases of AIDS on record in which the person seems to have recovered. While this number is small, it does suggest that even AIDS is not hopeless.

People with AIDS, regardless of how they contracted the disease, often feel guilty, lonely, and alienated, and suffer from poor self-esteem. Some of these feelings are supported by a society that limits access to school for children who have AIDS, argues about mandatory HIV testing, and wants health care workers to be prohibited from caring for the public if the worker is HIV positive. The message society sends is that people with AIDS have fewer rights than the rest of society, that they are less worthy than others, that they are bad people.

There is a dynamic tension between some parts of the HIV positive community, particularly the gay and lesbian groups, and other parts of society. The gay community has chosen to become politically active, working for civil rights of people with AIDS and increased research monies to find a cure for AIDS. The activism sometimes clashes with the conservative political values of others and each side offends the other. Healing in the gay community, including those with AIDS, requires dialogue in society. Moffat (1986) discusses a scene she witnessed between a gay man and a mother of an AIDS patient. The mother was trying to change her lifelong stereotypical view of gay people by attending a support group, listening to what was said, and sharing the pain of watching a son suffer. One young man in the group immediately assumed she must have been a bad mother, and told her she should be happy her son had people like himself to love him. This kind of polarization of viewpoints, blaming each other and assuming that each is bad for violating another's standard of behavior, does not help create relationship. It makes healing more difficult.

Self-righteousness by members of groups who feel morally superior to AIDS patients reinforces the patients' poor self-esteem and belief that they should withdraw from others. The new age thinker may convey the idea that wrong thoughts cause or at least support illness. Since the new ager does not have the disease, and the patient does, the message conveyed is one of "I'm better than you because I think right thoughts." Groups who promote the belief that AIDS (and other illnesses) are punishment from God also judge the victim, conveying the message that the person with the disease is bad. It must be remembered by health care professionals that many people who have no high-risk behaviors contract AIDS. To engage in thinking that suggests that those who do engage in high-risk behavior deserve the disease is to be judgmental and will interfere with any ability to establish and maintain a healing environment.

People with AIDS may blame themselves, parents, partners, society or their God figure for their disease. They need to experience forgiveness for their own guilt, and learn to forgive those others they feel contribute to their problems. They need to develop a connectedness with family and people who support and love them without bitterness or anger.

One of the characteristics of people who survive for a long time with AIDS is the sense of taking control of their lives. They refuse to be thought of as victims. They shop for a doctor who will give them the information they need without requiring treatments they do not want. They use anything they think will help: homeopathic remedies, laughter, vitamins, imagery, faith, hope, optimism, Therapeutic Touch and massage, a balanced diet, exercise, sufficient rest, positive prayer, and love. The nurse can help these people to create an environment in which they can thrive. Requirements for such an environment include:

- an intention to create a place of peace and healing
- people in the environment who are able to connect with those who may have a limited life span
- resources to assist in a search for meaning in life, including counselors, spiritual guides, literature on topics like meditation and retreat centers, and the willingness to talk
- willingness to turn inward, to examine self and identify one's strengths and resources
- creativity—murals on the walls that people can add to with colors or pencils, humor carts, and so on

Natural History

There is a natural history, a regular pattern to HIV infections, with some group and individual variations, according to the expert panel of the Agency for Health Care Policy and Research (El-Sadr et al., 1994). Infection occurs through blood or body fluids (sexual contact and blood transmission via dirty needles or contaminated blood products are the most obvious and common methods). There may be a stage of flu-like symptoms, followed by a period of seropositivity, but no symptoms. The symptomatic stage may occur as long as 10–14 years after the seropositive results are first known. This early stage may last several years before the advanced state of AIDS is experienced (Bouman, 1994). Thus, the person with AIDS may have had many years of living with positive HIV test results, and may have developed many skills and a lot of knowledge about the disease.

Long-term survivors of AIDS do not consider themselves victims. They take charge of their own healing. They have T4/CD4 counts monitored every six months while they are asymptomatic, and they understand that counts above 600 do not bring a recommendation for medication from the established medical community because there is no indisputable evidence that medication helps at this stage. There are so many side effects from the medications available that the physicians usually prefer to wait until a stage at which the medication has been shown to be effective. These survivors also know that T4/CD4 counts less than 500 indicate that antiretroviral therapy should be started, and counts should be monitored more often. Counts under 200 mean that prophylaxis for pneumocystic pneumonia should be started. Long-term survivors generally get the monitoring done, but they follow the medication recommendations selectively, depending upon the current knowledge of the AIDS community.

Many HIV positive people continually balance the information they receive from the medical establishment, the popular culture represented by on-line AIDS information services, health food stores and homeopathic practitioners, and the way they feel intuitively. The nurse should seek knowledge of current AIDS treatments and what AIDS patients, including those who are probably terminal within the next year, are doing for themselves. Self-treatment that is complementary to medical care will become a part of the treatment plan the nurse and patient establish together.

It is beyond the scope of this kind of book to describe the medical and nursing treatments for people with AIDS in all stages of the disease. However, for easy reference, table 10.1 lists the common antiretroviral medications and their side effects.

Medication	Adverse Effects
Zidovudine (ZDV) (formerly AZT)	granulocytopenia, anemia, nausea, headache, confusion, myositis, anorexia, hepatitis, seizures, nail discoloration
Didanosine (ddI) (Videx)	potentially fatal pancreatitis, peripheral neuropathy, nausea, diarrhea, confusion, seizures, and in children, peripheral retinal atrophy
Zalcitabine (ddC)	aphthous ulcers, esophageal ulcers, peripheral neuropathy, stomatitis, cutaneous eruptions, thrombocytopenia, pancreatitis

TABLE 10.1   *Common Antiretroviral Medicines*

From El-Sadr, W., Oleske, J. M., Agins, B. D., et al. (1994). *Evaluation and management of early HIV infection. Clinical practice guideline no. 7.* AHCPR Publication no. 94-0572. Rockville, MD: Agency for Health Care Policy and Research, Public Health Service, US Department of Health and Human Services.

There are a number of medical conditions that commonly complicate the clinical picture of AIDS. Among them are:

Candidiasis, esophagus, respiratory tree

Cytomegalovirus disease

HIV-related encephalopathy

Herpes simplex lasting more than a month

Kaposi's sarcoma in patients less than 60 years old

Leukoencephalopathy

Lymphoma, including Burkitts and immunoblastic

Pneumocystis carinii pneumonia

Salmonella septicemia

Wasting syndrome (Bouman, 1994)

Special problems that require assessment or screening by the nurse for people who are seriously ill with AIDS include:

1. respiratory conditions, which could indicate pneumocystic pneumonia or tuberculosis, two of the most common opportunistic HIV-related infections

2. oral lesions suggestive of herpes simplex, destructive periodontal disease, and other infections

3. eye problems, the most common of which is cytomegalovirus retinitis (CMV), which results in visual disturbances and vision loss

4. signs of sexually transmitted diseases, including neurosyphilis

5. Pap smears for women to detect invasive cervical cancer (El-Sadr et al., 1994)

More information about the care of patients with these conditions and the screening techniques and programs can be found in the AHCPR guidelines (El-Sadr et al., 1994).

Death due to AIDS is a different path than most deaths, because of the nature of the disease. Dementias may occur, making the patient difficult to deal with, and sometimes dangerous, as was the patient who crouched in a corner and threatened to stick the nurses with his I.V. needle if they approached.

Medication to restrain patients who develop combativeness due to dementia and sufficient help for the threatened staff, family, and others must be available. Safety, so that the patient does not unintentionally inflict harm to self or others, becomes an important consideration.

Other serious problems at the time of death for the AIDS patient include difficulty with pain control, skin breakdown because of severe wasting and weight loss, nutritional problems due to poor appetite and oral lesions, and fatigue and weakness. These problems are amenable to careful, planned, and adequate nursing care. If the nurse and those who are significant in the life of an AIDS patient have created a nonstigmatizing environment in which the physical care is combined with sensitive and compassionate concern for the relationships that exist, allowing for forgiveness, choice in the patient's treatment plan, release of anger, and love, the patient will live well until death.

VIOLENT DEATH

Death by one's own hand or the hand and intention of another touches friends, family, and the wider community in a unique way. Suicide and homicide are among the leading causes of death in adolescence. Both leave survivors who have difficulty in understanding why such a thing could have occurred and if something should have been done to prevent it. Survivors are often guilt ridden, though nurses should not assume that guilt is always characteristic.

Yoko

Yoko was 15 years old when her mother decided she should begin contributing to the family income by becoming a prostitute. Yoko was afraid of her first customer and believed that her new life would mean the death of the dreams she had for herself—college, marriage, and a family. So she jumped out of a sixth-floor window and died.

Yoko's mother grieved for her, but she had difficulty understanding Yoko's lack of respect for her family's wishes, though it was not something Yoko wanted for herself. Obedience was important to the mother, and she felt shame that her daughter did not do as she was told. The shame did not diminish her love for Yoko, but guilt was not her problem. Nurses who did not take the time to understand this could not understand why the mother did not feel guilty, and they judged her as an unfeeling, uncaring mother because she violated their belief about how mothers should act. The mother should have been afforded the same care in her grief as other mothers would have received—she should have been allowed to spend some time with Yoko's body to say good-bye, to express her grief to nurses if she wanted to do so, and she should have been given any personal effects of Yoko's that she wanted and that were not confiscated for legal purposes. To do otherwise was to render judgment on another person without all the facts.

Healing the dying, when the dying occurred unexpectedly as a result of suicide or homicide, requires helping to bridge the chasm that opens between the one who dies and the ones left behind. There has been no opportunity to prepare, to examine existential concerns or meaning in life and death. There may be multiple legal, financial, or social problems. The nurse may meet these survivors in many settings, as stress-related illnesses following this kind of family trauma are not uncommon.

Suicide

Suicide has been called "the cruelest death" (Lester, 1993). People grieving the death of someone whom they feel had a choice to live or die, feel betrayed, angry, puzzled, abandoned, rejected, ambivalent, and strange (Robinson, 1989). Family members may get little support from others, and sometimes ask for none, believing that the dead loved one forfeited a right to the kind of mourning that goes on for others. Religious ritual may be affected by the way the person dies, because some groups believe that suicide is a reason to deny burial in consecrated ground. This leads to isolation of the family from the support of that religious organization.

Parents sometimes become overprotective of other children if one child has committed suicide. Some children respond by engaging in risky behavior or losing self-esteem since they obviously can not replace the brother or sister who died and make the parents grieve less. They often feel guilty, believing that if they had fought less, been kinder, or acted differently, the sibling would be alive. They may have trouble understanding that the dead sibling is really dead. Nightmares, poor school work, and depression may follow. Parents may be unaware of these changes because of their own grief.

Friends of teens who commit suicide may be at risk for cluster or copycat suicides. Teens who have already lost a friend to suicide see dying together as glamorous and attention getting. While rare, it occurs often enough for schools to bring in special counselors when a teen commits suicide to prevent the tragedy of more teens following the pattern. Study of the Bergenfield tragedy, a cluster of four suicides by teens in one carbon monoxide-filled garage, showed that each of the four teens had problems previously (Dolce, 1992). Studies of other clusters confirm that teens do not commit suicide without thought, but suicide by a classmate or acquaintance may give them the idea of a glamorous way to solve some of their problems. Preventing suicide in this group depends on identifying troubled youths.

If a family has a history of problems, the nurse may make referrals to people who can monitor signs of risk of suicide. These signs include:

- suicide threats
- previous suicide attempts
- statements about wanting to die
- getting affairs in order
- giving personal treasures away
- personality changes that seem greater than the situation warrants

- withdrawal, apathy, lack of appetite, or other signs of depression
- attempts to isolate oneself
- hopelessness, helplessness, or worthlessness
- suddenly becoming calm or peaceful after a period of turmoil, especially if preceded by signs listed above (Robinson, 1989, p. 143)

Homicide

Homicide, death caused by the intention of one person to end another person's life, has the same characteristic of sudden, unexpected, and helpless end to a relationship, but there are some differences. If the murderer is known, as is often the case, the family may have divided alliances, conflict, and anger. Guilt is evident in most cases of family violence that ends in homicide.

If the victim was killed in a robbery or the killer is unknown for other reasons, relatives may also be in fear of their own lives. One young widow realized that her husband's killer, who was as yet unapprehended, had taken his address and house keys in the robbery. No one knew the reason for the murder. She was sure the killer would return to get her.

Healing for all these people begins when they find out about the loss and can begin in the place the victim is pronounced dead, often an emergency room. Like the parents of the child who dies of SIDS, friends and family of suicide or homicide victims may need to spend time with the body, and to take some memento of the one who died. When it is not possible to see the body, as in the case of fire when the body is not recognizable, being in the same building or area where the body is may be helpful. They need information about legal issues, like autopsy requirements and when results will be known. There needs to be a place for them to meet with the police so that they can get information regarding property, suspects, and other issues. Clergy, family, and other people involved need to be called, so access to a phone is helpful. An institution that sets up an environment in which these basic needs can be met is valued by the society it serves. Two women lost their husbands in a murder-robbery incident. The bodies were taken to two different hospitals for pronouncement of death. A few weeks later each new widow received a communication from the hospital to which her husband had been taken. The first widow opened the envelope and saw that she had received a bill for $75 for services rendered in the emergency room. The second widow opened the envelope and read a sensitively written letter expressing condolences for her loss, and offering referrals to grief counselors or hospital clergy. It is obvious that the second hospital, though also submitting a bill for services, is working to create a healing environment, and in this case, at almost no cost to the hospital. Nurses take the lead in initiating this kind of effort.

Societal Issues

Social values in the United States are changing rapidly, and attitudes toward violence are a part of that change. Violence is an epidemic, and homicide is a major cause of death, especially among young people, disproportionately so among black men. Increasing numbers of deaths of this kind move politicians and lawmakers to try measures like limiting the kinds of guns available to buy, increasing numbers of police on the streets, and providing more social programs to redirect young people to other kinds of life choices in handling anger and conflict.

Attitudes toward some kinds of suicide are changing, as well. Assisted suicide is becoming a political issue. The well-known Hemlock society and Americans Against Human Suffering both promoted legislation (in California and Washington) that would make it legal to help people voluntarily commit suicide under very rigid guidelines. In some cases, the Washington initiative would make it legal to request and receive active, voluntary euthanasia (Quill, 1993). Both referenda were defeated. In Michigan, Dr. Kevorkian was tried for helping people he said were terminally ill commit suicide. He has some popular support.

While society is in the process of defining values related to suicide and homicide, the survivors of victims of violence are confused and ambivalent. Support for the individuals is colored by an ever changing view of the acceptability of violence. Shooting a person to death seems to be acceptable if the victim is engaged in a robbery on the shooter's premises or is threatening him in some way. Suicide is somewhat acceptable (and so families can be supported openly) if the victim was terminal, but rarely if the victim was depressed. The degree of guilt experienced by the family varies in part according to societal mores. Families and friends, the grief-stricken, are confused.

One way people deal with this kind of confusion is to take a stand and work on societal issues from the viewpoint of a victim or a family of a victim. Socially helpful ways of dealing with anger and guilt include joining (or forming) victims' rights groups, grass-roots organizations for social change to help future generations avoid epidemics like the current violence. Examples of socially active groups that help in this way are Citizens Against Violence (CAVE), Families of Victims of Handguns, and People Against Rape (PAR). These and other groups provide a way to act out anger and change society in the direction a person believes it should go. Other people become politically active and work for specific legislation. Nurses, too, can use these groups to work for social change they feel is needed, and in doing so, work for healing of self and society.

THE DEATH OF A NURSE

When a nurse is terminally ill, other members of the health care team, and especially the nurses, are confronted by their own mortality in a very direct way. The dying nurse is a reminder of the fact that a caregiver is also human and is subject to the same rules of life and death as patients. For the nurse-caregiver who uses distance and separation from patients as a coping skill designed to protect from burnout and intense emotion, it may be impossible to care for a friend or other nurse. So the nurse who is dying may be separated from the nurses who had formed a support system in both personal and professional life.

Professional caregivers may also want to render extraordinary care. Larry Dossey, M.D. (1993) writes of being in bed with a back problem. Many of his professional friends came by to help him, but each had a different treatment or kind of care (like massage, imagery, and others) sure to help. In his case as in others, when a treatment is not chosen, the caregiver who offers it may feel rejected. A barrier may be created by loving people who cannot let the patient be in charge and accept the patient's choice of treatments. Caregivers have a hard time letting those they love make choices contrary to what they would have chosen. Healing the dying nurse, like healing other dying individuals, focuses on relationships and comfort. Barriers to the dying nurse getting the same care needed by any dying patient include:

- fear of asking for help from others due to fear of being labeled a difficult patient

- recognition of difficulty of caregivers coping with care of a dying patient

- concerns about confidentiality of information

- belief that the nurses are too busy with people who can be helped to a greater degree (a way of continuing to care for others, even when dying)

- inconsistent or sporadic teaching, the health care team believing that the dying nurse has information she does not have

- insufficient rest, too many visitors

A dying nurse is a special person, needing the same care as other dying patients, but in a different way. Nurses believe that they know how the dying nurse feels. As with all perception, it must be validated by clear communication with the dying one, or it may be inaccurate. Honesty, the ability to allow the dying person to make choices contrary to the ones the caregiver would choose, and sensitivity to needs for visiting or rest, information or ventilation are critical components of caring for a person who is important in the community of nurses.

NEAR-DEATH EXPERIENCES

Dying people who discuss their near-death experiences (NDEs) with the nurses often become special to the nurses who care for them because their stories are so unique. While the NDE may be either positive or negative to the person who experiences it, it usually helps the person to see meaning in life.

Some NDEs are not particularly dramatic. One police officer who was shot and being treated in a trauma center remembers floating above her body, watching the team cut off her clothes, and realizing how sick she was. But she immediately found herself back in her body, and in her fight to get well forgot the NDE entirely until a nurse asked her if she had experienced anything strange or unusual during her illness. Her NDE stimulated her to wonder what happened, to examine the seriousness of her illness, and to consider what happens after death. It did not change her life in any appreciable way, but it started her investigation into the meaning of her own life.

A dock worker who was in a near-fatal accident was also asked about unusual experiences, and broke down and began crying. He told of going through a dark tunnel, reaching a beautiful new land. In that bright and peaceful place, he saw and talked with white-robed figures and his dead mother. After several more experiences there, he returned to his pain-filled body and hoped to die so he could reenter the land. Once he was out of the intensive care unit, he told his wife of his experience, but he told no health care workers until the nurse gave him the opportunity. This man had a very emotional experience and was already planning how to change his life. His wife was supportive of the changes, which included church membership and a new interest in community activities.

Both of these patients believed they had come close to death and survived. Both verbalized that they no longer feared death, though the process of pain and separation from loved ones was still upsetting. Both of them needed to talk with someone who believed their unique experiences and could simply listen, without ascribing meaning beyond the incident. That is, the nurse neither glorified the incident, nor minimized it. The experience a person has when he comes close to death is not death itself. Therefore, one cannot support nor deny the concept of life after death as it was described by a person who has experienced an NDE. Life after death is a matter of faith, not science. The NDE suggests that there may be peace and much more than we understand at the moment of death, and it can be a comfort to families to know that a loved one has experienced such an event. Each experience is unique and has unique meaning to the person who experiences it.

Care of the person who has experienced an NDE includes:

- listening without judgment
- helping the person to share the story with family
- referral to clergy or spiritual guide if requested
- counseling, if the person is planning to change direction in life and that direction is contrary to the family's values
- introducing the person to others who have had the experience, if others are available, to form a small support group

Sometimes when caring for a person who is dying, the nurse hears the person relate the experience of becoming peaceful and no longer fearing death because of an NDE. If the family is not present when this occurs, the nurse has the opportunity to share the experience with them, and it often gives much comfort to them, to know that the person died in peace. Other visions the dying person may relate, like the presence of a dead family member, may be shared with family for whatever meaning they have to them.

SUMMARY

Every life is unique, every person special. This chapter is about people who are special because they are members of a particular group of people who require special care when they are dying. We care differently for people who are our family or friends, who are stigmatized or have diseases we fear, who are vulnerable, as children are, or who have special stories that help us to search for our own meaning in life. We care differently for their families and loved ones, because they have different needs.

Every nurse must take the time to know herself, to know if her own coping depends upon separating herself from dying friends or avoiding difficult situations. Every nurse needs to know if fear of AIDS or other disease interferes with the care of those who have the disease. Every nurse needs to be able to listen to and support the patient with unique deathbed experiences.

References

Akner, L. (1993). *How to survive the loss of a parent.* New York: William Morrow and Co.

Benoliel, J. Q. (1991). Multiple meanings of death for older adults. In E. M. Baines (Ed.) *Perspectives on gerontological nursing.* Newbury Park: Sage Publications.

Bouman, C. C. (1994). Nursing management of adults with immune disorders. In P. Beare & J. Myers (Eds.), *Principles and practice of adult health nursing* (2nd ed.). St. Louis: C. V. Mosby Year-Book, Inc.

Buckingham, R. (1990). *Care of the dying child.* New York: Continuum.

Corr, C. A., Fuller, H., Barnickol, C. A., & Corr, D. M. (1991). *Sudden infant death syndrome: Who can help and how.* New York: Springer Publishing Co.

Dolce, L. (1992). *Suicide.* New York: Chelsea House Publishers.

Dossey, L. (1993). *Healing words.* San Francisco: Harper.

El-Sadr, W., Oleske, J. M., Agins, B. D., et al. (1994). *Evaluation and management of early HIV infection. Clinical practice guideline no. 7* (AHCPR Publication No. 94-0572). Rockville, MD: Agency for Health Care Policy and Research, Public Health Service, U.S. Department of Health and Human Services.

Lester, D. (1993). *The enigma of adolescent suicide.* Philadelphia: The Charles Press, Publishers.

Moffat, B. C. (1986). *When someone you love has AIDS.* New York: NAL Penguin.

Quill, T. (1993). *Death and dignity: Making choices and taking charge.* New York: W. W. Norton & Co.

Robinson, R. (1989). *Survivors of suicide.* Santa Monica, CA: IBS Press.

White, R., & Cunningham, A. M. (1991). *Ryan White: My own story.* New York: Dial Books.

THOSE WHO CARE FOR THE DYING

CARING FOR DYING PEOPLE

Death overload is a term that indicates that a caregiver has experienced the death of too many patients in a short period or too much personal investment in patients for too long a time (Vachon, 1993). For nurses who started one palliative care unit, their distress scores were equal to those of newly widowed women and higher than those of women with newly diagnosed breast cancer who were undergoing radiation therapy. Yet in other studies, nurses who cared for people with life-threatening illnesses, including hospice nurses, had less distress and more coping skills than nurses in other fields. Some nurses clearly have the ability to grow into the role of caring for dying people in a way that supports their own growth and expert practice, and to change the environment so that it can support other caregivers to do the same. It is important for nurses who care for the dying to clearly understand the emotional risks to themselves and plan to use the experience to nurture their spirit and develop the ability to be present in each moment, savoring life in its fullest, and finding meaning in being there for the dying patient.

One Model of Occupational Stress

Vachon (1987) developed a model of occupational stress based on Antonovsky's definition of stress. Stress is "a demand made by the internal or external environment of the organism that upsets its homeostasis, restoration of which depends upon a non-automatic and not readily available energy-expending action" (Antonovsky, 1979, p. 162). In this model, stress is different from routine stimuli, and it is different for different people. Routine stimuli may become stressful if the balance of the environment is upset. One death on a nursing unit where death is a likely prognosis may be a routine stimulus. Several deaths in a day or a week may upset the environment of the unit, cause disruption in the ability of those present to hope, to plan for care, and to grieve sufficiently for each dying person.

According to Antonovsky, in order to reestablish the routine in this scenario, the nurses must take some action. For the nurses to go on as if nothing had happened means that the normal pattern of caregiving, the camaraderie, the gestalt of the unit will be adversely affected, morale will suffer, and death overload or burnout will occur among the staff. Vachon's model helps identify the areas of action that can help.

Simply stated, the occupational stress model explains that job stress is the consequence of the interaction of personal characteristics with the environment over time. To affect the consequences of job stress, including burnout or overload, one must act on either personal characteristics or the environment or both. Personal characteristics that influence the perception of an individual nurse, leading to an evaluation of the event as stressful include:

- age—younger nurses have developed fewer coping skills and see events as more stressful

- personality, including motivation for caring for the dying, personal value system, and coping style

- previous and current stressful life events, especially experience caring for dying people, both as a nurse and as a family member or friend

- social support from other professional colleagues, as well as from friends and family outside the profession

There are many motivations for caring for dying or otherwise vulnerable people. Each of these motivating characteristics can be a source of strength or a source of stress. Motivation for caring for the dying may come from a deep set of values demanding action on behalf of suffering people, perhaps as a call of faith, or a desire to improve the world. But if a nurse (or other health care provider) is motivated to care for the dying because of the unresolved death of a loved one, the nurse is particularly at risk. Other unresolved deaths are likely to lead to distress and burnout. A positive outcome would be that the stress itself becomes a motivating factor to resolve the family losses.

Hardiness is a personality characteristic that is helpful to patients and nurses alike. A hardy person has a sense of commitment, a sense of meaningfulness, physical/or psychological endurance, the power to influence events, boldness, and a feeling of challenge. Conversely, the person who is not hardy is alienated, powerless, threatened, and has little sense of goal directedness. Hardy nurses and hardy patients can work together by sharing control and decision making in planning care. These characteristics create a powerful impetus for individuals to create an environment or an atmosphere of healing.

A nurse's support system also influences the perception of burnout or stress following the death of one or more patients. If a nurse's support comes mainly from a social group, there may be a lack of understanding of the depth of his feelings about the events at work. In addition, his social group may not want to hear about sad or difficult times, may not want to provide the needed listening ear or be available to cry with the nurse who is sad. If the grief is a regular occurrence, friends get tired of hearing about it, though they are often willing to provide needed distraction. A group of professional people with whom the nurse can share the losses may be more helpful. They are more likely to understand, to have experiences that can be usefully shared, and to have coping skills that are helpful to the nurse who has lost a patient. They know when to recommend a different course of action like taking time off.

Other personal characteristics that leave the individual caregiver vulnerable to the particular stressors of caring for dying people include family variables. Birth order (the eldest child), gender (female in most cultures), and a family history of substance or other abuse predispose some people to continue their role of caregiver of the family in a professional role of caregiver. An eldest, female, adult child in a dysfunctional family is often attracted to a caregiving role, and any of the health care professions, like nursing, social work, physical therapy, and medicine provide that opportunity. A nurse who comes from a dysfunctional family may continue the dysfunctional behaviors of the family in professional life when stress is severe.

Environmental characteristics that predispose caregivers working in that environment to experience tension and poor coping skills related to stress include:

- poor communication patterns with other caregivers in the area, and with patients and their families
- role overload, role strain, and role ambiguity
- inadequate resources and staffing (adapted from Vachon, 1993)

Poor communication patterns not only predispose the nurse and others to the consequences of occupational stress, but have been documented to be harmful to patients (Baggs et al., 1993). For nurses, the inability to discuss patients adequately with physicians often means that they feel unable to get appropriate care for the patient, such as medication orders or other treatment. The physician may feel frustrated at not having the knowledge about the patient on which to base decisions, such as whether new medications are necessary. The other staff, therapists, personal care aids, and consultants all try to function without needed information. Professional rivalry develops. Team members form coalitions and factions begin to form, with conflict soon following.

Communication problems with patient and family are stressful because the patient may not be able to express need, so the team cannot meet that need. The family may blame the staff and physician for the patient's failing health. Ultimately, caring for this individual is not satisfying because it becomes constant conflict. The lack of trust between all parties is a source of conflict.

Role strain, overload, and ambiguity are all stressors with which nurses in many settings are familiar. Role strain occurs when one has difficulty performing all the required aspects of one's role. This may be related to lack of information, as when there are communication problems and all the relevant information is not available. Lack of knowledge about what to do or how to do it (as when pain control is inadequate, and one does not know what to do) may be a factor. Or lack of resources to complete the tasks or make the best choices for the care of an individual may be the cause of a nurse not performing all the aspects of the role satisfactorily.

Role overload occurs when one feels that there is just too much to do. Nurses tend to try to finish, no matter what the job, often staying late, charting after hours, and becoming frustrated and tired. This is particularly identified as stressful if it is required by others, not taken on willingly by the health care worker. For example, most nurses do not mind staying late because a patient needs to talk about a problem or there is a need to contact a doctor about a new order. But if the case load as assigned is consistently greater than safe staffing ratios permit, it is role overload, and leads to people feeling stressed.

Role ambiguity and role conflict are the result of not knowing what the role really involves, and what another person's role includes. This problem reflects the fact that the role expectations are not clearly defined in the system. Advanced nurse practitioners are prone to this kind of problem. A pain management specialist may be called for medication titration, education of staff in pain assessment, management of epidural medication systems, writing policies, presenting information to physicians, massage, and imagery. To do all of these things well is very difficult, and may lead to role overload, but without knowing what the expectations of the role are, it is hard to choose which of those tasks are most urgent, which are the priorities. Role conflict is experienced when the individual's many roles in life conflict, as when one's professional life conflicts with personal goals. An example occurs when one is asked to be on call during a time when the family has been promised an outing.

The fear of inadequate resources is related to the current health care financing crisis, and it is a reality in some health care settings. There is always a dynamic tension between the provision of high-quality care, which requires resources, and the need to restrain costs in health care, which have been rising much faster than inflation for many years. Limited dollars do not automatically mean that care will be substandard. Unfortunately, when resources are limited, staff is often limited, and psychosocial care is sacrificed. For the dying patient, that is a critical aspect of care, and nurses feel care is substandard if it is not available. Professional health care providers in any discipline who cannot provide the kind of care they believe is important, especially to people with terminal illness, are going to experience the consequences of job-related stress.

Consequences of Stress for Providers of Care

Stress-related problems, like the causes of the stress, are related to the system, the individual, or both. Coping mechanisms used to handle stress-related problems are those things one does to make the system supportive to staff and those things one does to care for self.

One young nurse tearfully turned in her resignation to her supervisor after the death of the third patient that week. She told the supervisor that she could not cope with death, that she could not sleep, eat, or stop thinking about one of the patients. This nurse was sure she could have done more for all of them, especially one who died unexpectedly. She felt "so sorry for the three-year-old who lost his mother" that she bought him a stuffed rabbit, then could not give it to him. Her spiritual distress was becoming all-consuming.

This nurse exemplified many consequences of stress. Caregivers of dying people reexamine their own belief systems, sometimes suffering an existential crisis of faith. They grieve each loss, and if the losses come too quickly, they do not complete their grieving before the next death. Other common feelings include:

- guilt
- anger
- irritability
- frustration
- helplessness
- inadequacy
- sleeplessness
- depression

These feelings may lead to problems with interactions with patients, family, and other staff. To cope with increasing pressure, this nurse admitted that she had avoided contact with new patients, reasoning that the patients she knew needed her more. Intellectualizing her actions in this way reinforced her feelings of inadequacy, since she knew her assessments were not complete, and she did not work toward establishing the trust that newly diagnosed, terminally ill patients needed. She avoided meaningful contact with individual patients by making rounds with other staff, or while the patients were asleep. Her judgment suffered, omitting referrals that were obviously needed, making others that were not. All of this reinforced her sense of guilt, and she became evasive with her coworkers, flaring in anger when asked to stay late. Her fiance resented her constant funereal conversation, wanting to know when she would begin to laugh again. Finally, she agreed with him that resignation was the way out of the dilemma. Results of the feelings experienced by nurses who are not coping well with the deaths of patients may include clinical problems like:

- avoiding the patient
- poor clinical judgment
- unrealistic expectations
- staff absences
- outbursts of anger
- lack of anticipatory planning
- staff conflict
- scapegoating
- interdisciplinary power struggles
- staff fatigue
- ambivalence toward patients

Two things need to happen for the young nurse to grow in her ability to care for the dying and to find satisfaction, even joy, in doing so. The first is that she learns to care for herself. The second is that the environment, including the institution or organization she is associated with and people she works with, becomes energetic, supportive, and healing.

CHANGING THE ENVIRONMENT

Leadership skills are required to change the environment. Policy and politics are not bad words, and the ability to use them is necessary for change to happen. Politics is defined here as: to gain and use enough power to get done what needs to be done. This may mean forming coalitions with other groups of caregivers to make policies that work. For example, one group of nurses was having difficulty getting the anesthesia team to respond quickly when called for pain management. Instead of complaining to each other and becoming frustrated by the situation, they carefully documented the time lag between calls to the service and response for a month. They presented their information to their supervisor (called an outcomes manager in that system) who was responsible for quality assurance. That manager gave the information to three attending physicians who regularly admitted patients to that special care unit. At the same time, the nurses on the unit had developed reasonable goals for response time and a policy that set out a plan by which nurses could get help when needed for patient pain management, who was responsible, and what to do if the team did not respond. A team meeting between the anesthesia team, attending physicians, a patient advocate (ombudsman), and nursing representation quickly adopted the policy change. The anesthesia team began responding within defined time limits, and when one of them did not, the policy as adopted was used and the anesthesia department intervened to provide the help the nurses needed to provide care. This is an example of the appropriate use of politics—forming coalitions between members of various groups to change policy to meet defined goals.

Another leadership skill is the ability to recognize when staff ideas have merit and should be supported, even if resources are scarce. Staff may recognize when support groups of various kinds are needed, and when they have become routine and outlived their usefulness. In either case, the ability to begin programs like support groups and discontinue them when they have served their purpose should be a clinical decision, and policy should not make those decisions difficult to carry out. Nurse managers can support initiative and change, helping staff who have ideas with merit to implement them.

Team building is another skill nurse managers use to create an environment of healing. Nurses who care for the dying sometimes need an extra day off, help in caring for a difficult patient, or other considerations. Some nurses should not be assigned to a certain kind of patient based on feelings related to family history. For example, a nurse may be unable to care for a burn patient if a family member was in a fire and there are unresolved feelings about that incident. Consideration for assignment change and an occasional mental health day are ways of recognizing unique needs of staff members.

Nurse colleagues need to know and accept the fact that each of them will need that consideration and be willing to provide it for others. That willingness to stand in for colleagues only comes if the members of the staff who work together trust each other to use requests for help only when needed. Most staff members will become resentful of another member of the staff who:

- asks for help with every difficult patient

- takes time off from work for family convenience

- does not make an effort to resolve the problems that put up barriers to caring for some patients

- requests special consideration more often than seems indicated

A needy staff person will become isolated and possibly disruptive to the rest of the staff, calling in sick more often and in other ways attempting to meet needs for self-care that interrupt the flow of the team effort to create a special environment.

Team building requires that all members of the team agree on a few basic principles. The first is to decide who the members of the team are. The nursing team (whether a home care group, a hospice group, a hospital group, or other) is a team nested within a larger organization, and the whole health care team should have an identity. The whole team should have a sense of purpose, of goals that are shared, and how those goals will be met. A mutual respect for other team members and their abilities is a prerequisite to a trusting relationship and the ability to leave a task in another person's hands. Members of different professions sometimes have overlapping competencies. That is, a nurse, a clergyperson, and a social worker may all have skill in counseling a patient regarding an identified spiritual need. But if they all try to counsel one patient, that person may be confused or refuse the ministrations of one or two members of the team, leading to hurt feelings. It is better for the team members to recognize the abilities of each other, have a plan for deciding who does what (including the patient's choice), and trust that the person doing the work can do it well. If the care provider does not request help with the task, the other care providers do not attempt to intervene (or rescue the team member) even if they think they could do it better. While there are times when a knowledgeable person can suggest alternate ways of approaching a problem, criticizing the person entrusted with the care of the patient often creates distrust and conflict. Offering to help is acceptable if the environment as a whole is supportive to the workers, and the offer is not likely to be viewed as interference or distrust. The team may agree that there are many right ways to do something.

Fostering an atmosphere of mutual support makes it possible for all the staff to put into words their feelings about the care they give and the people for whom they care. Regular team meetings allow problem solving for patient care issues, as well as the identification of problems staff members may be developing in relation to that care. The well-functioning team can point out to the stressed nurse what seems to be happening so that the nurse can assess the situation and move to change it. Or the team may offer to take on some responsibility for care if overload is a contributing factor. The group may help each other understand why a particular patient makes them angry or makes them feel guilty. Sometimes an outside support person, like a visiting psychologist or a psychiatric consultation liaison nurse, may help the group dynamics, so the team does not become negative.

A mutually supportive environment is one perceived by patients and staff as a healing environment. Such an environment is built on trust, recognition of the skills and abilities of colleagues, a leadership that can accomplish appropriate change and attract needed resources, and the establishment of a kind of unique gestalt, or special feeling about the place and its people. That special feeling is easy to recognize, hard to define. People in such environments greet each other (and strangers) warmly, often with smiles. Though incredibly busy, they are not short tempered or sour in demeanor. There is a frequent use of humor, but not dark humor that risks offending people. People are able to laugh at their situations, sometimes even at the physical changes in themselves. Family and visitors soon pick up the feeling. There are instances of a whole group of people (not usually staff) arriving at the room of a person who has lost all hair due to treatment with their heads shaved in a show of support. Staff members can laugh with the group, encourage the camaraderie, have the group visit other bald patients, and join in the fun.

These environments are also creative. No two are alike. The main feelings are caring, serenity, and love. There is an intention to help other people, a desire to make a difference. There is a clear sense of purpose. That is expressed in spontaneous conversations—begun with a statement like, "How shall we help Mrs. K?" Patients feel free to ask for the help they need. The healing environment for the nurse includes policies that support the ability to take a day off when needed, or to arrange for a group meeting for the purposes of sharing care problems and frustrations. The ability to get a facilitator for the group can be helpful.

The physical environment is both stimulating and serene, accomplished by having things like plants, colorful pictures, music of different types at different times, balloons when celebrating, and quiet when peace is needed. Personal items belonging to both staff and patients may be present. For staff, the items may be pictures on walls, helpful books, photographs of previous patients, awards, or other remembrances. For patients, photographs and personal items with special meaning are there. People get together in small groups. Some people spontaneously hug others, and those who do not like to hug shake hands or receive a pat on the back as a more acceptable way to make physical contact. In some settings, a separate room is available for private conversations, meditation, and prayer, a private telephone, reading materials, special rituals, or crying.

Healing environments can be found in places like the waiting room of an intensive care unit, the outpatient department of a large urban hospital, nursing centers for primary care, hospice units or organizations, or specialty care settings, like transplant units or oncology centers. When they exist, both patients and nurses are able to experience healing.

CARING FOR SELF

Wise, mature, expert nurses root their care for others in healthy life patterns for themselves. They have knowledge of their strengths and self-confidence in their abilities. They have confronted their own mortality, and have developed a philosophy of life that is compatible with the choice they have made to work with dying people. The death of a patient is not viewed as a failure. They see each moment in life as an opportunity to make choices of some kind, for good.

Keegan (1994) suggests that the most important category of attributes of healers, including nurses, is attitude, since it is from attitude that people act. That attitude is grounded in a sense of meaning and purpose in life, a sense of becoming empowered by service to others, a sense of one's place in the natural world, and an ability to use one's life experiences (even the sad ones) in the care of others. Nurses who do this are recognized by their joy, caring spirit, clear sense of purpose, and intent to use hands, heart, and spirit. They are hands-on, empathetic, genuine, centered, and connected people.

Motivation

The question Why care for people who are dying? is important. For each nurse to become a healer of the dying, identifying motivation is important. Occasionally a nurse who has been caring for the terminally ill for some time has a sudden realization that caring for these people is an attempt to answer questions for himself about difficult instances in life. The nurse must identify the fact that unresolved issues in life can be barriers to care and to happiness and joy in the work. When the nurse realizes that unresolved problems exist, it is important to confront those issues in a useful way by requesting the help of a professional person, a competent spiritual guide, or a knowledgeable colleague who has the expertise to help.

A second nurse may be professionally challenged by the many ways available to help dying people both in physical care for comfort and for care beyond the physical that involves search for meaning and peace. This nurse may be passing through the palliative care model, later using skills learned from the lessons the dying have to teach with other patients who may not be dying. This nurse is intellectually stimulated by palliative care.

Another nurse in the same area revels in the growth of each patient as that person comes to terms with the nature of mortality and the beauty of life in many forms. This nurse is a nurturer, a person who is likely to use a creative approach to care to help people achieve their own goals. This nurse may also care for the dying as a manifestation of service to humankind, a spiritual calling to be fulfilled, intrigued and compelled by each individual's search for meaning in life.

Yet another nurse may find joy in the physical care of very ill people, using a variety of techniques found to be effective in the care of dying people, like massage, yoga, breathing exercises, Therapeutic Touch, and others. This nurse probably cares for herself in a similar way, taking classes in aerobic exercises or T'ai Chi, maintaining an active life-style.

The motivations for each of these nurses are not mutually exclusive. The nurse-healer strives for balance, growing in all of life by understanding how his feelings influence his actions with patients. This nurse learns new and useful skills of communication. He learns systems of exercises and comfort measures. He actively maintains his physical health to help sustain energy and hardiness. This nurse also works to develop a rich spiritual life, maintaining connections with his inner self and the larger universe. A healer may focus on one area for a while, then move to a different level of growth as a result of an experience with a dying patient.

Coping Techniques

Coping skills include anything one can use to alter the relationship between the person and the environment to change the negative results of psychophysiologic consequences of stress. Ted is an example of using forgiveness as a means of coping with a set of feelings that had been negative in his life for years.

Ted

Ted was an RN with four years of experience on a general medical hospital unit. Patients on the unit had a variety of serious diagnoses, and many of them died. One patient reminded Ted of an aunt who had died when he was five years old. That was also the age when he began school. The death of his aunt became linked with the abandonment he felt when his parents left him at the school door. Venting his feelings about the patient to a supervisor, Ted suddenly realized that the onset of his poor job performance (which he had labeled as burnout) was related to his feelings about this past experience. He decided to talk over how he felt with his parents, and to tell himself he forgave them for the perceived abandonment. This simple insight and related action helped Ted to consider forgiveness as an important conscious way to deal with hidden grudges and negative feelings about others. This gave him a new way of relating to other staff, and brought him new joy in his work. He worked on letting go of bad feelings about others by simply forgiving them, without regard to assigning blame. Forgiveness for Ted became a coping mechanism.

There are a number of techniques that help nurses who are caring for dying patients stay healthy. Maintaining their balance between a philosophy that helps to give meaning to what they are doing and growing in ability to confront personal challenge is one goal. Continuing the kind of connection with others that leads to service is another.

Maintaining health is the first important coping technique nurses use to combat the special stressors of caring for the dying. There are many physical strategies used to enhance the health of both nurses and patients who feel stressed. Obviously, good nutrition and weight control, regular exercise, adequate sleep, and sufficient resources to maintain these things are important.

Vigorous exercise is helpful because it contributes to good weight control and helps develop strength and endurance. Exercise initiates biochemical changes that support one's ability to feel tranquil and peaceful after the exercise, and provides a time to be away from the source of the stressor. A regular schedule of well-chosen exercises that are both physically challenging and pleasurable is most likely to be continued over time.

Other kinds of physical activities that are useful coping strategies include massage, diaphragmatic breathing, and distraction. Each of these techniques must fit into a program of general time management, valuing time for self as well as competent, planned patient-care time management. Massage is a technique used for many years by nurses for patients. But at least one nursing department invested in a massage chair for staff! Nurses knowledgeable in massage techniques help each other with periodic 15-minute neck and shoulder massages. Release of muscle tension in shoulders and back breaks the feeling of stress, refreshes, and relaxes. Time is scheduled, allowing nurses to anticipate a period of focus on themselves. The brief time of focus on the caregiver in a practical, caring way reinforces a caring environment and gives the nurses a respite in an otherwise busy day of focus on others.

Diaphragmatic breathing is a useful technique to learn for relaxing and to begin the centering process. Consciously realizing the path each inhalation takes through the respiratory passages, and allowing each breath to move to the bottom of the respiratory tree by moving the diaphragm downward and outward moves the whole person toward feeling more relaxed. As the slow, long exhalation occurs, a person feels shoulders moving downward and tension slowly leaving the body. To help with stress at work, a nurse should practice diaphragmatic breathing at home, in either a supine or sitting position. Putting one's hand on the abdomen is an easy way to know if the abdomen is involved in the breath, or if shallow, tense breaths are a pattern. Once a pattern of abdominal breathing is the norm, the nurse can think words like, "I can feel this way whenever I take a deep breath and cross my fingers." Connecting the relaxed feeling to the physical act of crossing fingers (or any other physical cue) helps the body to remember how it feels to relax. A nurse who regularly practices this technique has the ability to break the cycle of stress and muscle tension identified even at the bedside of a dying patient in just a few seconds. The pattern is:

- recognize the feeling of tension
- take an abdominal breath
- use a physical cue that has been practiced
- allow shoulders to sag and relaxation to be experienced during the exhalation

This technique, or pattern, is useful by itself to help relax for a few minutes or to lead to more profound states of relaxation. For the nurse who is attempting to help the patient by using Therapeutic Touch or some other energy work, breathing from the diaphragm helps to become focused. It helps a nurse to move to a place of peace within, an awareness of the space created between patient and nurse that is healing to both people in this unique relationship. Diaphragmatic breathing may also be a way of centering, or an adjunctive technique to other forms of relaxation, including:

- progressive muscle relaxation (PMR)
- autogenic relaxation
- sentic cycles
- relaxation imagery
- meditation in many forms

Nurses who practice diaphragmatic breathing for a time often go on to learn other relaxation techniques that become a consistent resource for dealing with stress and tension. Practice sessions should occur at least three times a day, for five to ten minutes a session. Within a week or two, the skill will be learned. With continued practice, the ability to relax will deepen. Relaxation is defined in table 11.1.

Distraction is another coping technique, which is necessary to break a pattern of tension, to get away from an intense situation if only for a few seconds. Humor, a deep breath, a massage break, someone's story about a family member or a book recently read, or a lunch break can serve as a useful distraction,

Progressive muscle relaxation

Alternately tensing and relaxing skeletal muscles, starting with the feet and going through each major muscle group. Concentration is on feeling the difference between a tense and a relaxed muscle group. The tension phase is omitted when one is comfortable in knowing what relaxation feels like.

Autogenic relaxation

Mentally repeating phrases scripted to reflect the sensations of a relaxed body, such as "Each muscle is relaxed and limp."

Sentic cycles

Mentally rehearsing a series of intense emotions, alternating opposite emotions, such as peace with anger.

Imagery

Using an internal process, the imager explores various senses, such as vision, auditory, kinesthetic, and other senses.

Meditation

An inner process of listening to that which is inside oneself and which connects with the universe. Depending upon the type of practice, meditation can be a relaxation technique, an altered state of consciousness, a hypometabolic state, or a spiritual practice, such as contemplative prayer or a type of yoga.

***

TABLE 11.1   Relaxation Techniques Defined

allowing the nurse to come back to the situation with a fresh viewpoint and perhaps more energy. A heavy work schedule should not be used as an excuse to avoid a lunch break. While it may be necessary to make a meal a short one, it is most often true that a nurse who has been away from an intense situation for a few minutes is able to return feeling more able to help. Family members, too, need to be encouraged to take a break, or a deep breath, or tell a story now and then to decrease the tension in the environment.

If a long, intense relationship comes to an end through the death of a favorite patient or someone for whom it has been a significant challenge to care, the distraction may need to be longer, perhaps a day off or a vacation to rest and refresh one's spirit. Planning to use that time as fun, scheduling things that are not reminders of a patient or death and dying may be important, and may be alternated with the need to grieve and remember significant people, including patients, in one's life.

DEVELOPING THE SPIRITUAL SELF

Knowing that one's life has meaning and confronting one's mortality are the key elements in developing the ability to care for people who are dying. A nurse who has not identified a reason for being does not have direction in life and a framework for action. It is easy to get distracted from any sense of purpose, pulled from a moment of joy into someone's problems, another's loss, a third person's fears. *Healing the dying* means healing oneself by forming connections with the Universe and all that it is. It means a path one can count on, a way one travels with confidence, accompanied by others for parts of the journey.

One Tired Nurse

Samantha was tired, frustrated, and felt like being alone. She decided her spirit was tired and needed renewal. Life seemed hard. She planned a weekend retreat at a monastery that offered guest cottages and quiet gardens in which to walk. During the weekend, the Catholic monks invited this Protestant woman (the only woman on the grounds) to their regular services. Samantha accepted, thinking the music would assist her search for peace. She was surprised when they offered her a seat in the choir (the section of pews where the monks sit). When the monks went to the altar for communion services, she stayed in her seat, knowing that the rite was reserved for those of the Catholic faith. One of the monks came to her and said, "Why don't you come with us, just for a hug." Suddenly, her spirit soared. Seeking a weekend of solitude and peace, she found a community with a spirit that resonated with hers. They were united in a mutual caring, the beauty of the place, the music, and God. Samantha does not need to return to the monastery to feel the joy and to know there is a bridge between the present and the unseen.

A search for meaning need not be a lonely search, a sad or intellectual search. In fact, learning to listen is the most important requirement. The use of quiet, peaceful environments like gardens or meditation rooms is useful for quieting the chatter of the mind, hearing the whisper of nature, of the inner self, and connecting to one's own spirituality. A structure or discipline of some kind is useful, for it provides landmarks by which to gauge progress. For example, people who grow up regularly attending religious services have gone through consistent rites of passage, moving to new religious education classes each year, having ceremonies indicating movement toward adulthood (like confirmation of faith, public expression of conversion, bar mitzvah), and joining groups of like-minded people on the search. When the inner development does not keep pace with the group's development, a person is likely to drop out, sometimes returning later. Inner development is supported by studies, the culture or religious group, and group and individual reflection on faith.

For some people, organized religion is not the road to a sense of connection with meaningfulness and purpose. Sometimes they attain an abiding spiritual focus by connections with nature. A walk along the oceanfront, a long hike in the mountains, or a meditative session next to a waterfall all provide a sense of oneness with nature and a knowledge of belonging to the community of humankind and the Universe. One's purpose is in being.

Whether one seeks a spiritual awakening within a group or as an individual, the path is an inner process. Whether one achieves a transforming moment, a peak experience always to be remembered, or proceeds through the process a little at a time, learning through each contact with each person, there is a growing sense of unity and purpose in being. One belongs here. One has a mission, a service. One is committed to a path of action.

There are many ways one can choose to develop a deeper spirituality or an ability to listen to the inner self. Other than formal association with a spiritual group, they include:

- learning to meditate or pray

- creating an environment that supports peace—using nature, music, or sounds like waterfalls or ocean waves, art or furniture, like a kneeling bench, or cushions to sit on

- reading literature that teaches how to develop a spiritual path, and biographies of those known for their spiritual natures
- setting a regular time to practice whichever form of discipline one chooses
- keeping a spiritual journal, or diary
- sharing one's journey with other spiritually mature people
- guiding other people in spiritual journeys
- enjoying life

SUMMARY

All people who care for terminally ill patients are at risk for developing a special kind of distress related to many losses and incomplete understanding of the role. They also have the potential for developing a life of service leading to great joy, a feeling of professional and personal competence, and an ability to live their own lives to the fullest. It is a matter of choice.

The person who chooses to grow through the experience of caring for others actively maintains a balance between all areas of good health: exercise, nutrition, sleep, social support, deepening friendships, commitment, and a clear sense of a spiritual journey, a connection with all of life through all generations. An understanding of one's meaning in life leads to the ability to enjoy it. Those who enjoy it can share it.

References

Antonovsky, A. (1979). *Health, stress and coping.* San Francisco: Jossey-Bass.

Baggs, J. D., Ryan, S. A., Phelps, C. E., Richeson, F., & Johnson, J. E. (1993). Collaboration in critical care. *Heart & Lung, 21*(1), 18–24.

Keegan, L. (1994). *The nurse as healer.* New York: Delmar Publishers.

Vachon, M. L. (1987). *Occupational stress in the care of the critically ill, the dying and the bereaved.* New York: Hemisphere.

Vachon, M. L. (1993). Emotional problems in palliative medicine: patient, family and professional. In D. Doyle, G. Hanks, & N. MacDonald (Eds.), *Oxford textbook of palliative medicine* (pp. 577–605). Oxford: Oxford University Press.

Epilogue

Ms. F. left the V.A. Hospital to go to school. Two weeks after she left, she was eating breakfast and reading the paper. Mr. Bower popped into her memory, and she wondered how he was doing. She remembered how he waited for her each evening, so often with a small issue, no really transcendent moments, nothing dramatic or memorable. Yet through the eight-month period that she had known him, he had changed. They had developed a special relationship that was satisfying and healing for each of them at different times. She remembered how he had helped when Luke died, giving up his room, and later telling her that she did well, helping her self-confidence and her sense of competency in her work.

He continued to question, to learn, to help his comrades, to become more settled and satisfied with life. He knew he would die, fought it for a time, and became progressively more peaceful. He had learned that he did not want to give up and would continue to do what he could to live well. He made peace with his God and with his family. He also made many plans. He made a will and left his medals to his newly found grandson. He shared this news with the men on his unit, and they rejoiced with him. He knew he had made a difference in life, that his life had meaning because of his wartime contributions. He had learned to be satisfied with his life, glad he had lived it.

Then Ms. F. read the small headline. It said, "P. Bower, war hero, dies of cancer." The notice went on to say he had died the night before. It listed his daughter and her family as next of kin. And there was a paragraph about his silver star and his heroism in saving lives of others.

Ms. F. had not realized the extent of his heroism. After a few moments of grief and sadness, she smiled. His life was closed, but he had taught her how it was to die. She felt he left more of a legacy than he realized as her teacher, and she was glad. It had been a healing relationship.

1 | Dosing Data for Pain Medications*

*From Acute Pain Management Guideline Panel. (1992). *Acute pain management: Operative or medical procedures and trauma. Clinical practice guideline* (AHCPR Publication No. 92-0032). Rockville, MD: Agency for Health Care Policy and Research, Public Health Service, U.S. Department of Health and Human Services.

Drug	Approximate Equianalgesic		Recommended Starting Dose (adults more than 50 kg body weight)		Recommended Starting Dose (children and adults less than 50 kg body weight)[1]	
	Oral Dose	Parenteral Dose	Oral	Parenteral	Oral	Parenteral
Opioid Agonist						
Morphine[2]	30 mg q 3–4 hr (around-the-clock dosing)	10 mg q 3–4 hr	30 mg q 3–4 hr	10 mg q 3–4 hr	0.3 mg/kg q 3–4 hr	0.1 mg/kg q 3–4 hr
	60 mg q 3–4 hr (single dose or intermittent dosing)					
Codeine[3]	130 mg q 3–4 hr	75 mg q 3–4 hr	60 mg q 3–4 hr	60 mg q 2 hr (intramuscular/subcutaneous)	1 mg/kg q 3–4 hr[4]	Not recommended
Hydromorphone[2] (Dilaudid)	7.5 mg q 3–4 hr	1.5 mg q 3–4 hr	6 mg q 3–4 hr	1.5 mg q 3–4 hr	0.06 mg/kg q 3–4 hr	0.015 mg/kg q 3–4 hr
Hydrocodone (in Lorcet, Lortab, Vicodin, others)	30 mg q 3–4 hr	Not available	10 mg q 3–4 hr	Not available	0.2 mg/kg q 3–4 hr[4]	Not available

[1]**Caution:** Doses listed for patients with body weight less than 50 kg cannot be used as initial starting doses in babies less than 6 months of age. For recommendations, consult the *Clinical Practice Guidelines for Acute Pain Management: Operative or Medical Procedures and Trauma* section on management of pain in neonates.

[2]For morphine, hydromorphone, and oxymorphone, rectal administration is an alternative route for patients unable to take oral medications, but equianalgesic doses may differ from oral and parenteral doses because of pharmacokinetics differences.

[3]**Caution:** Codeine doses above 65 mg often are not appropriate due to diminishing incremental analgesia with increasing doses but continually increasing constipation and other side effects.

[4]**Caution:** Doses of aspirin and acetaminophen in combination opioid/NSAID preparations must also be adjusted to the patient's body weight.

Dosing Data for Opioid Analgesics

Levorphanol (Levo-Dromoran)	4 mg q 6–8 hr	2 mg q 6–8 hr	4 mg q 6–8 hr	2 mg q 6–8 hr	0.04 mg/kg q 6–8 hr	0.02 mg/kg q 6–8 hr
Meperidine (Demerol)	300 mg q 2–3 hr	100 mg q 3 hr	Not recommended	100 mg q 3 hr	Not recommended	0.75 mg/kg q 2–3 hr
Methadone (Dolophine, other)	20 mg q 6–8 hr	10 mg q 6–8 hr	20 mg q 6–8 hr	10 mg q 6–8 hr	0.2 mg/kg q 6–8 hr	0.1 mg/kg q 6–8 hr
Oxycodone (Roxicodone, also in Percocet, Percodan, Tylox, others)	30 mg q 3–4 hr	Not available	10 mg q 3–4 hr	Not available	0.2 mg/kg q 3–4 hr[4]	Not available
Oxymorphone[2] (Numorphan)	Not available	1 mg q 3–4 hr	Not available	1 mg q 3–4 hr	Not recommended	Not recommended
Opioid Agonist-Antagonist and Partial Agonist						
Buprenorphine (Buprenex)	Not available	0.3–0.4 mg q 6–8 hr	Not available	0.4 mg q 6–8 hr	Not available	0.004 mg/kg q 6–8 hr
Butorphanol (Stadol)	Not available	2 mg q 3–4 hr	Not available	2 mg q 3–4 hr	Not available	Not recommended
Nalbuphine (Nubain)	Not available	10 mg q 3–4 hr	Not available	10 mg q 3–4 hr	Not available	0.1 mg/kg q 3–4 hr
Pentazocine (Talwin, others)	150 mg q 3–4 hr	60 mg q 3–4 hr	50 mg q 4–6 hr	Not recommended	Not recommended	Not recommended

Dosing Data for Opioid Analgesics (continued)

Drug	Usual Adult Dose	Usual Pediatric Dose[1]	Comments
Oral NSAIDs			
Acetaminophen	650–975 mg q 4 hr	10–15 mg/kg q 4 hr	Acetaminophen lacks the peripheral anti-inflammatory activity of other NSAIDs
Aspirin	650–975 mg q 4 hr	10–15 mg/kg q 4 hr[2]	The standard against which other NSAIDs are compared. Inhibits platelet aggregation; may cause postoperative bleeding
Choline magnesium trisalicylate (Trilisate)	1000–1500 mg bid	25 mg/kg bid	May have minimal antiplatelet activity; also available as oral liquid
Diflunisal (Dolobid)	1000 mg initial dose followed by 500 mg q 12 hr		
Etodolac (Lodine)	200–400 mg q 6–8 hr		
Fenoprofen calcium (Nalfon)	200 mg q 4–6 hr		
Ibuprofen (Motrin, others)	400 mg q 4–6 hr	10 mg/kg q 6–8 hr	Available as several brand names and as generic; also available as oral suspension
Ketoprofen (Orudis)	25–75 mg q 6–8 hr		

[1]Drug recommendations are limited to NSAIDs where pediatric dosing experience is available.
[2]Contraindicated in presence of fever or other evidence of viral illness.

Dosing Data for NSAIDs

Drug	Usual Adult Dose	Usual Pediatric Dose[1]	Comments
Magnesium salicylate	650 mg q 4 hr		Many brands and generic forms available
Meclofenamate sodium (Meclomen)	50 mg q 4–6 hr		
Mefenamic acid (Ponstel)	250 mg q 6 hr		
Naproxen (Naprosyn)	500 mg initial dose followed by 250 mg q 6–8 hr	5 mg/kg q 12 hr	Also available as oral liquid
Naproxen sodium (Anaprox)	550 mg initial dose followed by 250 mg q 6–8 hr		
Salsalate (Disalcid, others)	500 mg q 4 hr		May have minimal antiplatelet activity
Sodium salicylate	325–650 mg q 3–4 hr		Available in generic form from several distributors
Parenteral NSAID			
Ketorolac	30 or 60 mg IM initial dose followed by 15 or 30 mg q 6 hr Oral dose following IM dosage: 10 mg q 6–8 hr		Intramuscular dose not to exceed 5 days

Dosing Data for NSAIDs (continued)

Haight's Life Review and Experiencing Form

Childhood

1. What is the very first thing you can remember in your life? Go as far back as you can.

2. What other things can you remember about when you were very young?

3. What was life like for you as a child?

4. What were your parents like? What were their weaknesses, strengths?

5. Did you have any brothers or sisters? Tell me what each was like.

6. Did someone close to you die when you were growing up?

7. Did someone important to you go away?

8. Do you ever remember being very sick?

9. Do you remember having an accident?

10. Do you remember being in a very dangerous situation?

11. Was there anything that was important to you that was lost or destroyed?

12. Was church a large part of your life?

13. Did you enjoy being a boy/girl?

Adolescence

1. When you think about yourself and your life as a teenager, what is the first thing you can remember about that time?

2. What other things stand out in your memory about being a teenager?

3. Who were the important people for you? Tell me about them. Parents, brothers, sisters, friends, teachers, those you were especially close to, those you admired, those you wanted to be like.

4. Did you attend church and youth groups?

5. Did you go to school? What was the meaning for you?

6. Did you work during these years?

7. Tell me of any hardships you experienced at this time.

8. Do you remember feeling that there wasn't enough food or necessities of life as a child or adolescent?

9. Do you remember feeling left alone, abandoned, not having enough love or care as a child or adolescent?

10. What were the pleasant things about your adolescence?

11. What was the most unpleasant thing about your adolescence?

12. All things considered, would you say you were happy or unhappy as a teenager?

13. Do you remember your first attraction to another person?

14. How did you feel about sexual activities and your own sexual identity?

Family and Home

1. How did your parents get along?
2. How did other people in your home get along?
3. What was the atmosphere in your home?
4. Were you punished as a child? For what? Who did the punishing? Who was "boss"?
5. When you wanted something from your parents, how did you go about getting it?
6. What kind of person did your parents like the most? The least?
7. Who were you closest to in your family?
8. Who in your family were you most like? In what way?

Adulthood

1. What place did religion play in your life?
2. Now I'd like to talk to you about your life as an adult, starting when you were in your twenties up to today. Tell me of the most important events that happened in your adulthood.
3. What was life like for you in your twenties and thirties?
4. What kind of person were you? What did you enjoy?
5. Tell me about your work. Did you enjoy your work? Did you earn an adequate living? Did you work hard during those years? Were you appreciated?
6. Did you form significant relationships with other people?
7. Did you marry?

   (yes) What kind of person was your spouse?

   (no) Why not?
8. Do you think marriages get better or worse over time? Were you married more than once?

9. On the whole, would you say you had a happy or unhappy marriage?

10. Was sexual intimacy important to you?

11. What were some of the main difficulties you encountered during your adult years?

   a. Did someone close to you die? Go away?

   b. Were you ever sick? Have an accident?

   c. Did you move often? Change jobs?

   d. Did you ever feel alone? Abandoned?

   e. Did you ever feel need?

Summary

1. On the whole, what kind of life do you think you've had?

2. If everything were to be the same would you like to live your life over again?

3. If you were going to live your life over again, what would you change? Leave unchanged?

4. We've been talking about your life for quite some time now. Let's discuss your over-all feelings and ideas about your life. What would you say the main satisfactions in your life have been? Try for three. Why were they satisfying?

5. Everyone has had disappointments. What have been the main disappointments in your life?

6. What was the hardest thing you had to face in your life? Please describe it.

7. What was the happiest period of your life? What about it made it the happiest period? Why is your life less happy now?

8. What was the unhappiest period of your life? Why is your life more happy now?

9. What was the proudest moment in your life?

10. If you could stay the same age all your life, what age would you choose? Why?

11. How do you think you've made out in life? Better or worse than what you hoped for?

12. Let's talk a little about you as you are now. What are the best things about the age you are now?

13. What are the worst things about being the age you are now?

14. What are the most important things to you in your life today?

15. What do you hope will happen to you as you grow older?

16. What do you fear will happen to you as you grow older?

17. Have you enjoyed participating in this review of your life?

*Form copyrighted by Dr. B. Haight, College of Nursing, Medical University of South Carolina, Charleston, SC 29425-2404. Reprinted with permission.

NOTE: Derived from new questions and two unpublished dissertations:

Falk, J. (1969). The Organization of Remembered Life Experience of Older People: Its Relation to Anticipated Stress, to Subsequent Adaptation and to Age. (Unpublished Doctoral Dissertation, University of Chicago).

Gorney, J. (1968). Experiencing and Age: Patterns of Reminiscence Among the Elderly. (Unpublished Doctoral Dissertation, University of Chicago).

3 | Hot Lines and National Resources

HOT LINES

The following list of organizations maintain (at the time of publication) hot lines as indicated. This list was chosen for relevancy to the care of dying patients, and is not comprehensive. Current phone numbers can be found in any library that has a directory of 800 numbers or a current edition of *Lesko's Info-Power* by Matthew Lesko*. Or the National Health Information Clearinghouse can give current phone numbers. Call 1-800-336-4797 or Directory Assistance at (area code) 555-1212.

A useful tool for health care professionals is the *Health Hotlines* booklet available through the National Library of Medicine. It is a compilation of organizations with toll-free telephone numbers. It is free. Most are also listed in DIRLINE, NLM's on-line directory of information services for those who have access to the Internet or library facilities (see reference below).

Government

Health and Human Services—Social Security Administration:
    Information on survivor, disability, Medicare,
    or Social Security benefits   1-800-234-5772

Health and Human Services—
    Health Care Financing Administration:
    Referral service for second surgical
    opinions   1-800-638-6833

Health and Human Services—
    National Institutes of Health, National Cancer Institute:
    Cancer information and publications   1-800-4-CANCER

National Health Information Clearinghouse:
    For ordering publications on health and some
    referrals; e.g., for laser surgery experts   1-800-336-4797

National Library of Medicine:
    Information and reference database searches, 1913 to
    1970, including audiovisuals (Current searches should
    be done on-line through local library services and
    interlibrary loan programs)   1-800-272-4787

U.S. Department of Health and Human Services:
    Health information and referral service   1-800-336-4797

Private

American Cancer Society:
    Information, publications, referrals, support groups
    (local groups may offer equipment and other
    kinds of help)   1-800-ACS-2345

American Kidney Fund:
    Information, publications, financial
    assistance   1-800-638-8299

American Liver Foundation:
    Information and referrals   1-800-223-0179

American Sudden Infant Death (SIDS) Institute:
    Clinical research, educational offerings, and
    treatment facilities   1-800-232-SIDS

Children's Hospice International:
    Referral network   1-800-242-4453

Eldercare Hotline:
    Referrals to local resources nationwide   1-800-677-1116

Hospice Education Institute Hospicelink:
Referral network   1-800-331-1620

Joseph and Rose Kennedy Institute of Ethics
National Reference Center for Bioethics Literature:
On-line searches of database on bioethic
research (free)   1-800-MED-ETHX

National AIDS Hot Line (funded by Center for Disease Control):
AIDS information hot lines maintained in English,
Spanish, and for the hearing impaired   1-800-342-AIDS

National AIDS Information Clearinghouse:
AIDS publications, posters, databases,
and videos   1-800-458-5231

National Hospice Organization:
Referral and information help line
on hospices   1-800-658-8898

National Sudden Infant Death Syndrome (SIDS) Foundation:
Publications, information, and referrals   1-800-221-SIDS

Suicide and Rape 24-Hour Emergency Services
of the Humanistic Mental Health Foundation:
Crisis hot line, residential treatment program, and
financial assistance   1-800-333-4444

NATIONAL RESOURCES

The national resource agencies and organizations listed here are clearinghouses or referral points to help an individual find the help needed. This list is not comprehensive, but is limited to some of those agencies with the ability to help dying people. Addresses are given, but often a phone call brings quicker results. A few numbers are provided here.

A first call to the National Health Information Center at 1-800-336-4797 should be made to get the current phone number of the agency or hot line needed. Or you can call directory assistance in the area of the agency at (area code) 555-1212.

Bureau of Health Professions
Health Resources and Services Administration
5600 Fisher's Lane, Room 8-05
Rockville, MD 20857

Services: Maintains the National Practitioner Data Bank, which contains information on all disciplinary actions and malpractice claims or actions against licensed health care practitioners.

Centers for Disease Control (CDC)
Information Resources Management Office
Mail Stop C-15
1600 Clifton Road, NE
Atlanta, GA
1-404-332-4555

Services: A voice information system with prerecorded messages on health issues, with the ability to transfer the caller to a public health professional for more information.

Medical Care Ombudsman Program
Bethesda, MD
1-301-657-0404

Services: Free assessment of treatment options from a volunteer panel of top doctors.

National AIDS Information Clearinghouse
P.O. Box 6003
Rockville, MD 20850

Services: Free publications, posters, and videos about AIDS; a fact sheet, guidelines for the prevention of the spread of AIDS in school and at work; and The Surgeon General's report on AIDS. There are two databases for on-line search.

National Health Information Center
P.O. Box 1133
Washington, D.C. 20013
1-800-336-4797

Services: Publications and information resources on most health topics. Referral and current phone numbers of any of the National Institutes of Health and hot lines available. This number should be called first to check for current 800 numbers.

National Library of Medicine
8600 Rockville Pike
Bethesda, MD 20894

Services: Interlibrary loan; access to MEDLARS (Medical Literature Analysis and Retrieval System), an on-line database search system. MEDLARS provides access to other databases, like AIDSLINE, TOXLINE, CHEMLINE, HEALTH, CANCERLIT, SIDLINE, and others. This is the world's largest research library, and regional libraries will provide reference services and access to the National Library of Medicine.

National Second Surgical Opinion Program
Health Care Financing Administration
330 Independence Ave., SW
Washington, D.C. 20013

Services: Referral to physicians for second opinion, and pamphlets to help patients ask the right questions.

Public Information Division
National Institutes of Health (NIH)
Room 305
Bethesda, MD 20892
1-301-496-4143

Services: Free catalog listing publications available from each of the Institutes, addresses and phone numbers.

*Lesko, M. (1994). *Lesko's info-power* (2nd ed.). Detroit, MI: Visible Ink Press.

I N D E X

Note: Boldfaced page numbers reference information contained in figures and tables.

A

Acquired immune deficiency syndrome (AIDS), 185–190
Acupressure, pain control and, 88–89
Acupuncture, pain control and, 86
Acute pain, treatment guidelines, 91
Adaptive coping, 98
Addiction, pain treatments and, 81
Additives, pain control and, 80
Adjuvants, pain control and, 80
Advanced directives, 151–155
Advocacy, families and, 147–149
Affiliative faith, 120
Agency for Health Care Policy and Research, **164**, 187
AIDS, 185–190
American Cancer Society, 171
Americans Against Human Suffering, 194
Antiretroviral medicines, **188**
Anxiety, 98
  reducing, 110–116
    humor, 113–115
    life review, 115–116
    visualization, 111–113
Art
  death and, 9–11
  pain and, 92–93
Autogenic relaxation, **217**
AZT, **188**

B

Behavioral interventions, pain control and, 90–92
Bereavement, defined, **26**
Breakthrough pain, 76

Burkitts lymphoma, HIV-related, 189

C

Candidiasis, 189
Caregivers
  caring for self and, 212–217
    coping techniques, 213–217
    motivation for, 212–213
  characteristics of, 202–204
  environment, changing, 208–211
  spiritual development, 218–220
  stress,
    consequences of, 206–207
    occupational model, 201–206
  team building, 209–210
CAVE (Citizens Against Violence), 195
Children
  death of, 179–181
  pain and, 76–77
Chronic pain, described, 80–81
Citizens Against Violence (CAVE), 195
Clarification of information, described, 107
Clients, law and, 149–155
Cognitive interventions, pain control and, 90–92
Cohabitating couple, 32
Comfort
  assessment of, 50–53
    components for, **51**
  defined, 47–48
  mobility and, 60–62
  needs, 483
  quality of life and, 48–50
  resources aiding, 62–63
  sleep and, 56–60

touch and, 64–66
  whole person and, 53–55
    choice and, 54–55
    environment and, 55
    presence and, 53–54
    surveillance/safety and, 54
Commitment, defined, 132
Commune, 32
Communications
  fear and, 102–103, 105–108
  silence and, 107–108
  stress and, 204
Coping
  assessment of, 101–102
  discussed, 98–101
  patterns of, 99
  techniques, 213–217
Cytomegalovirus disease, 189

D
ddc (Zalcitabine), **188**
ddl (Didanosine), **188**
Death: The Final Stage of Growth, 27
Death
  art and, 11–12
  of children, 179–181
  language and, 9–11
  of nurse, 195–196
  overload, defined, 201
  of parents, 175–179
  peaceful, 20–21
  rituals and, 12–14
  siblings and, 182–183
  of spouse, 183–184
  sudden infant death syndrome (SIDS),
    181–182
  symbols and, 9–11
  technologic, 18
  see also Mortality
Depression, defined, **26**
Developmental theory
  dying/healing and, 27–28
  family, 33–34
Diaphragmatic breathing, as coping technique,
  215–216
Didanosine (ddl), **188**
Discomfort, described, 47
Distraction, as coping technique, 216–217
Drugs, administration of. *See* Medications,
  administration
Dying
  caring for, 201–207
  fears of, 97

healed, described, 3
occupational stress model and, 201–206
psychiatric illness in, 116–117
relationships and, 5–6
resources for,
  finding, 158–160
  governmental, 161–165
  need for, 157
  nongovernmental, 165–171
  referrals, 160–161
spiritual help for, 133–135
theories related to,
  family, 31–39
  grief, 26–31
  self-transcendence, 39–41
Dysfunctional grief, 30
Dyspnea, mobility assessment and, 61

E
Electrical stimulation, pain control and, 87–88
Emotional cutoff, defined, 141
Empathy, discussed, 132
Encephalopathy, HIV-related, 189
Endorphins, 78
Enkephalins, 78–79
Environment
  comfort and, 54
  nurses, changing, 208–211
Euthanasia, 194
Exercise, as coping technique, 215
Experienced faith, 120
Extended family, 32

F
Faith, types of, 120
Families
  connecting of, 141–149
    advocacy and, 147–149
    truth telling and, 142–146
  death in,
    children, 179–181
    parents, 175–179
    siblings and, 182–183
    spouse, 183–184
    sudden infant death syndrome (SIDS),
      181–182
  fears of, 97
  goals and, 139–141
  law and, 149–155
Families of Victims of Handguns, 195
Family, systems theory, 35–36
  approaches to, **33**
  developmental, 33–34

family types and, 32
grief and, 36–39
structural/functional, 34–35
systems theory, 35–36
Fear
communications and, 102–103, 105–108
coping with, 100
assessment of, 101–102
problem of, 95–96
reducing, 110–116
humor, 113–115
life review, 115–116
visualization, 111–113
support groups and, 108–110
types of, 96–98
Foot massage, pain control and, 88
Forgiveness, spirituality and, 126

G
Gate-control theory of pain, 78
Genograms, described, 37–38
Governmental resources, for the dying, 161–165
Grief
characteristics of, 28–29
children's, 177–178
consequences of, 29–31
definitions of, 26–27
dysfunctional, 30
family theory and, 36–39
parent's death and, 177
stages of, compared, **28**
theory of, 26–31

H
Haight's Life Review and Experiencing Form
(LREF), 115–116
Hand massage, pain control and, 88
Hardiness, as personal characteristic, 203
Healing
described, 3
palliative care and, 7–8
as relationship, 4–6
theories related to,
family, 31–39
grief, 26–31
self-transcendence, 39–41
Health care professionals, fears of, 97
Hemlock Society, 194
Herpes simplex, HIV-related, 189
Homicide, 193–194
Homosexual union, 32
Hope, spirituality and, 127–128

Hospice
discussed, 166–170
enrollment criteria, 168
responsibilities,
registered nurse, **170**
social worker, **169**
Humility, discussed, 132–133
Humor, fear reduction and, 113–115
Husband, death of, 183–184
Hygiene, sleep, 59–60

I
ICOI (Intravenous continuous opioid infusion),
83–84
Illness, stigmatizing, 184–195
Imagery, as relaxation technique, **217**
Industrial revolution, mortality,
after, 16
prior to, 15
Information
receiving, 105–106
responding to, 106–108
Insomnia, defined, 56–57
Intravenous continuous opioid infusion (ICOI),
83–84

K
Kaposi's sarcoma, HIV-related, 189
Kin network, 32

L
Language, death and, 9–11
Law, patients and, 149–155
Leukoencephalopathy, HIV-related, 189
Life review, reducing fear with, 115–116
Living wills, 151–152
Loss, defined, **26**
LREF (Haight's Life Review and Experiencing
Form), 115–116
Lymphoma, HIV-related, 189

M
Maladaptive coping, 98–100
Marriage family, 32
Massage, pain control and, 88
Meaning, spirituality and, 129–130
Medications
administration,
intravenous continuous opioid infusion
(ICOI), 83–84
nerve blocks, 84–85
oral, 82–83
patient-controlled analgesia (PCA), 84

rectal, 83
spinal anesthesia, 84–85
sublingual, 83
timing of, 82
transdermal patch, 83
sleep disturbance and, 58, 59
Meditation, 133
as relaxation technique, **217**
Memory, sustaining, 53
Mind, spirit and, 122
Mobility, 60–63
assessment of, 61–62
resources aiding, 62–63
Modal age of death, 19
Mortality
industrial revolution to World War II, 16
minority groups and, 14–15
post World War II, 16–18
pre-industrial revolution, 15
at present time, 19–20
see also Death
Motivation, self, 212–213
Mourning
defined, **26**
period, 27
Movement
comfort and, 60–63
assessment of, 61–62
resources aiding, 62–63

N

Narcotics, respiratory depression and, 81
National Cancer Institute (NCI), 163
National Hospice Organization, 167
National Institute of Mental Health (NIMH), 163
National Institutes of Health (NIH), 163
National Interfaith Coalition on Aging (NICA), 121
NCI (National Cancer Institute), 163
Near-death experiences (NDEs), 196–198
Nerve blocks, 84–85
NICA (National Interface Coalition on Aging), 121
NIH (National Institutes of Health), 163
NIMH (National Institute of Mental Health), 163
Noninvasive pain control, 86–87
Nuclear family, 32
Nurses
characteristics of, 202–204
death of, 195–196
environment, changing, 208–211
self care,
coping techniques, 213–217

motivation, 212–213
spiritual development, 218–220
stress,
consequences of, 206–207
occupational model of, 201–206
team building, 209–210

O

OARS Multidimensional Functional Assessment Questionnaire, 51, **52**
Opiates, treatment of pain with, 81
Oral medication administration, 82–83
Our Lady's Hospice, 166
Owned faith, 120

P

Pain
acute, treatment guidelines, 91
assessment of, 72–77
breakthrough, 76
child's, 76–77
chronic, 80–81
control flow sheet, **75**
creative arts and, 92–93
defined, 70–71
electrical stimulation and, 87–88
gate control theory of, 78
interview concerning, 72–73
massage and, 88
perception of, 79
problem of, 69–70
rating scales, 73–76
theories of, 77–79
transmission of, 77–79
treatment,
acupuncture and, 86
addiction and, 81
methods of, 82–92
nonpharmacologic, 85–92
pharmacological, 78–85
timing of, 82
Palliative care
defined, 7
healing and, 7–8
PAR (People Against Rape), 195
Parenthood family, 32
Parents, death of, 175–179
Patient-controlled analgesia (PCA), 84
Patients, law and, 149–155
Patient Self-Determination Act, 151
PCA (Patient-controlled analgesia), 84
People Against Rape (PAR), 195
Period of mourning, defined, 27

Physical stimulation, pain control and, 88–89
PMR (Progressive muscle relaxation), 91
Pneumocystic carinii pneumonia, HIV-related, 189
Prayer, 133
Presence, comfort and, 53–54
Procreation family, 32
Progressive muscle relaxation (PMR), 91, **217**
Psychiatric illness, in dying, 116–117

Q
Quality of life, comfort and, 48–50

R
Rectal medication administration, 83
Referrals, making, 160–161
Reflection, described, 106–107
Relationship, healing as, 4–6
Relaxation techniques, 90–92
defined, **217**
Religion, spirituality and, 123–124
Resources
for dying people,
finding, 157–160
governmental, 161–165
need for, 157
nongovernmental, 165–171
referrals, 160–161
Respiratory depression, narcotics and, 81
Rituals, death and, 12–14
Role
ambiguity, 205
overload, 205
strain, 204–205

S
Safety, comfort and, 54
Salmonella septicemia, HIV-related, 189
Scars, effects on relationships, 4–5
Searching faith, 120
Self motivation, 212–213
Sentic cycles, **217**
Shiatsu, pain control and, 88–89
Siblings, death and, 182–183
SIDS (Sudden infant death syndrome), 181–182
Silence, communications and, 107–108
Single parent family, 32
Sleep, 56–60
assessment of, 57–58
hygiene, 59–60

Social Security Administration, **164**
Spinal anesthesia, 84–85
Spirit, mind and, 122
Spiritual
distress, 125–130
defined, 125
nursing interventions, 131–135
health, 121–122
need, 125–130
self, developing, 218–220
Spirituality
assessment of, 130–131
development of, 120–121
forgiveness and, 126
hope and, 127–128
meaning and, 129–130
nature of, 119–120
religion and, 123–124
trust and, 128–129
Spouse, death of, 183–184
St. Christopher's, 166
treatment in, 167
Stress
consequences of, 206–207
interpersonal communications and, 204
occupational model of, 201–206
Structural/functional family theory, 34–35
Sublingual medication administration, 83
Sudden infant death syndrome (SIDS), 181–182
Suicide, 191–193
Support groups, fear and, 108–110
Surgery, pain control and, 86
Surveillance, comfort and, 54
Sustaining memory, described, 53
Symbols, death and, 9–11

T
Team building, 209–210
Technologic death, 18
TENS (Transcutaneous electrical nerve stimulator), 87
Theories, usefulness of, 25–26
Therapeutic touch (TT), pain control and, 89–90
Touch, comfort and, 64–66
Transcendent moment, 40
Transcutaneous electrical nerve stimulator (TENS), 87
Transdermal patch medication administration, 83
Trust, spirituality and, 128–129
Truth telling, within families, 142–146
TT (Therapeutic touch), 89–90

V

Veterans Administration, resources from, 162–164
Violent death, 190–195
Visualization, fear reduction and, 111–113

W

Wake, defined, 13–14
Wasting syndrome, 189

Wife, death of, 183–184
Wills, living, 151–152
World War II, mortality,
    after, 16–18
    prior to, 15–16

Z

Zalcitabine (ddC), **188**
Zidovudine (ZDV), **188**